The Office Workout:
75 Exercises to do at Your Desk

by Kent Burden

Contents

This book is dedicated to my wife Maria who tirelessly tests my programs for the workplace, making sure that my crazy ideas actually work!

This book is also dedicated to my grown children Kellen and Sydney, who help me navigate the world of social media and technology with humor, patience and creativity.

And last but not least, this book is dedicated to our cats, Goober and Daisy who keep me from sitting for prolonged periods of time, because every time I come back to my chair, they are sitting in it; and to our dog Inkadoo who insists on regular strolls around the block so I can practice what I preach.

1
Introduction

Let's take little a trip through time. In 1840, 69 percent of all American jobs were in agriculture. These jobs were hard physical labor. Workers did tasks like baling hay, plowing fields, milking cows and raising barns, which kept Americans lean and mean. A pedometer study of an Old Order Amish community (these guys are still pretty much living like our 1840 ancestors) revealed that the average Amish man logged 18,000 steps a day (a little over nine miles) and the women logged 1,400 steps (about seven miles) while performing the basic tasks of everyday living.

But by the 1950s everything had changed. Our economy had morphed into a service and industrial economy with 50 percent of the jobs being in the service sector (office, and customer service) and 40 percent of the jobs being in the industrial sector (factory and manufacturing jobs). Most of these jobs were far less physically intense than the agricultural jobs but still required a great deal of physical effort. The office in the 1950s was actually a fairly active place as office workers spent their days typing letters on manual typewriters, making copies on mimeograph machines that had to be hand cranked, bustling around filing documents in big file cabinets that were far away from their desks, and other semi-active duties. Inner-office communication mostly depended on getting up and going to somebody else's desk on your own two feet. If you had to research a topic, you headed to the nearest public library and searched the shelves for the book that held the information you needed, and climbing a ladder to get that book on the top shelf and slogging around with a stack of heavy books was not uncommon. Industrial jobs tended to be even more physical than service jobs, although not as physically demanding as agriculture. In 1950, 33 percent of U.S. adults were overweight and 9.7 percent were clinically obese.

Fast forward to today. More than 75 percent of all jobs in America are in the service sector, fewer than 20 percent are in the industrial sector, and less than 5 percent are in the agricultural sector. Today technology has pretty much sucked all the activity out of our everyday lives. Remember that pedometer study of the Old Order Amish community? Well today's average American takes just 5,000 steps a day (about 2.5 miles). Even worse, most of the things that kept people active in the 1950s office have been eliminated in today's office. Typing is a breeze with keyboards that register your key stroke with the lightest of touches (if you've ever used an old manual typewriter you know what I'm talking about). Need to put that report in your files? Just hit a few keys and that file is stored in the cloud.

Making copies is just as easy and most of us never need to leave our chair to get them since we all have a printer/copier on our desk within easy reach. Got to tell Lisa in accounting about the change of venue for this afternoon's meeting? Just send her an email and while you're at it, forward the receipt for the ink you ordered online for your printer. Time to get started on that big presentation you have next week? Better Google the stats on manufacturing trends and create a killer power point presentation for the Skype meeting with China. You can do all of this without ever standing up. You don't even need to leave your desk to meet face to face with the clients in China who also don't need to leave their desk to meet with you. The average American sits for a whopping 11 hours a day. Most of us are virtually chained to our chairs! Is it any wonder that in 2013, 69 percent of Americans are overweight and 35.1 percent are clinically obese? Not only is all that sitting making us fat, it's also making us sick. The rise in lifestyle diseases like diabetes, heart disease, stroke, kidney disease and certain forms of cancer are now being linked to prolonged sitting. Heck it's even making your back hurt.

What we really need is to put movement back into our daily lives, and since most of us spend a lot of our day at work, that's the first place we need to start. This book is about bringing more activity to your daily life in an effort to improve your overall health. The "side-effects" of doing this simple program are weight loss, increased energy, better mental focus, improved productivity and creativity.

2
What is this Office Workout Thing?

The Office Workout? You're probably thinking this is crazy talk. Nobody works out at work; when you're at work you…well…work. You know, create spread sheets, make sales calls, do customer service, write code or whatever it is they pay you to do. Working out is not on the list. Exercising might take you away from your work which could get you fired. Besides, who wants to be all sweaty and out of breath at work? No, you're probably thinking that it's best to put the whole idea of working out at work out of your head.

But what about that article you read in the Huffington Post that said spending long hours doing little or no physical activity (which pretty much sums up most of your days at work) can cause heart disease, diabetes, kidney disease, obesity and some forms of cancer? That's pretty scary stuff. Even worse is the segment you may have seen on ABC News illustrating that doing 30 to 60 minutes of sustained exercise isn't enough to undo the damage that sitting for long periods of time does to your health. Developing some terrible disease doesn't sound like a great idea; getting cancer or having a heart attack would probably keep you out of work, which probably wouldn't make your boss very happy. And then there was that article in the New York Times…*The New York Times* for Pete's sake, citing new research that said if you were 45 years old or older and sat for 11 hours a day you were 40% more likely to die in the next 3 years than people who sat for only 3 hours a day. You know that you sit a lot more than 3 hours almost every day. Maybe this *Office Workout* thing is not such a crazy idea after all.

So what should you do?

In this book, I'm going to show you how to workout at your desk without breaking a sweat or getting out of breath, and even better, it won't take you away from your work duties because all of the exercises will be done for very short periods of time (1-5 minutes) right at your desk. Because working out at work is different than working out at home or at the gym, you will need to be respectful of your fellow employees, adhere to a simple code of conduct and make your micro workouts fit into your daily work life. I will also discuss why being more active over the course of the day is such a powerful tool for better health and how it may actually be a more effective tool for weight loss than the old school way of working out. After that we will throw in "ultra low-intensity cardio" that you do while you work and the technology and equipment you'll need to make this program super effective and make you more productive at work than you've ever been. I give you a 10 Super-Secret Bonus Exercises No One Will Know You Are Doing at Your Desk.

Last but certainly not least, I will give you 75 exercises broken up into three sections for easy-to-do micro-workouts that will help you strengthen your entire body, engage your postural muscles and improve the health of your back and pack a big wellness punch. *The Office Workout* will change your health for the better, help you lose weight, make you look and feel better and maybe even lengthen your life! Now let's get you up and out of your seat and on the road to a healthier you. What the heck are you waiting for? Let's get started!

3
Getting the Ball Rolling

Before we get started there are a couple of things you need to do. First, before starting this or any other exercise program you should consult with your personal health care provider to be sure that the exercises contained in this book are right for you and your current state of health.

Second and equally important you should talk to your boss about what you're planning to do and get his or her approval. This is not something you want to try to do on the down-low-- you know, sneak it in when you think no one is looking and be all 007 about it. That's the kind of thing that could get you fired. Not only that but it's just not ethical. Your company has rules and policies that you agreed to when you signed up to work there and it's only right to abide by those rules and policies. The truth of the matter is there are a lot of great benefits for you in doing this program and a lot of great benefits for your employer if they let you do this program. To support you in your effort to improve your health I have created a chapter that you can show to your boss to explain why you should be allowed to workout at work and why letting you do that will actually benefit the company in terms of productivity and money savings (and those money savings can be significant!). Heck if you're enterprising, savvy and smart, you could set up a company-wide program, save the company a ton of money and maybe even get a promotion!

As you start down this road to a more active everyday lifestyle, we need to keep in mind that this is new territory we're exploring and the things we did in the old territory won't work here. **Specifically, you can't work out at work in the same way you might work out in the gym or at home.** So let's lay down a few rules. I guess this makes me the "Miss Manners" of the office workout world.

- **Don't Sweat It:** I know working up a sweat is pretty much the point when you go to the gym, but not at the office. Huge armpit stains and a sweat soaked blouse or dress shirt is just plain gross and smelling like Lance Armstrong after he climbed the Pyrenees Mountains in the Tour deFrance isn't going to win you any friends in the office. What we're doing is ultra low intensity exercises which have their own health benefits, so leave that gym mentality behind.
- **Silence is Golden:** I've spent a large portion of my life in the gym environment and the one thing I've noticed is that people make the weirdest noises when they workout. Grunting, groaning, whistling, panting or shrieking is not going to go over very well in the office environment. If you're doing this office workout thing correctly almost no one notices.
- **Jimmy, that's something you do in your "*Private Time*":** That's right. Never start doing your exercises in front of clients, customers or guests. Doing a couple of minutes of exercise in front of your fellow employees is fine but never in front of the people who bring the company revenue.
- **Timing is Everything:** In order to get the benefits of this work you only need a few minutes each hour so don't abuse the privilege. If your boss is forward-thinking enough to let you do this, then make sure you show him or her they made a good decision.

- **Safety First:** Make sure any equipment you use is in good working order and secured appropriately and be sure to put it away after you use it. A resistance band or a set of hand weights left on the floor of your office or cubicle can be a disaster waiting to happen.
- **Work it out:** Many of the things we'll be doing can be done while you work but if you need to make a decision between finishing your workout or finishing your work …then work it is!

If you follow these simple guidelines, your personal health, your job, and your fellow employees can live in harmony.

4
The Benefits

There are tons of benefits to being physically active and these benefits go well beyond just what traditional exercise can do for your body. The new science of sedentary studies is now showing that things most of us wouldn't consider to be "exercise" at all, if done regularly during the day, can have amazing health benefits. Finally there are the benefits that can be gained by your employer if they support and encourage all of their employees to be more active over the course of the day. The potential cost savings is staggering! (More about that later)

Physical Benefits of Exercise

Let's start with what most of us think of as exercise. Regular "exercise" (running, biking, strength training, playing sports, stretching, etc.) can improve bone health, creating stronger healthier bones and lowering your risk of osteoporosis; it can improve lung function and increase lung capacity, improving oxygenation to all the cells of the body; it can improve muscle tone and muscle strength; it can help maintain and improve muscle and joint flexibility. It can also help lower stress levels by increasing "soothing" brain chemicals like serotonin, dopamine, and nor epinephrine. Many people already know that.

What's really amazing though is that according to a 2010 study from the University of California, San Francisco, exercise may actually work on a cellular level to reverse the toll of stress on our aging process. Researchers found that stressed-out women who exercised vigorously for an average of 45 minutes over a three day period had cells that showed fewer signs of aging compared to women who were stressed and inactive. Working out also helps us to mentally let go of things that are troubling us "by altering blood flow to those areas in the brain involved in triggering us to relive these stressful thoughts again and again," says study coauthor Elissa Epel, an associate professor of psychiatry at UCSF. Exercise also has some other surprising benefits for brain health. Research suggests that by doing high intensity exercise (burning at least 350 calories) at least 3 times a week, you can reduce symptoms of depression as effectively as if you were taking antidepressants.

Exercise can also improve your ability to learn. Exercise increases the level of brain chemicals called "growth factors" which help make new brain cells and establish new connections between brain cells to help us learn. Complicated activities, like playing tennis or taking a dance class, provide the biggest brain boost. You're challenging your brain even more when you have to think about coordination, explains one researcher.

According to the Alzheimer's Research Center, exercise is one of the best weapons against the disease. Exercise appears to protect the hippocampus, which governs memory and spatial navigation, and is one of the first brain regions to succumb to Alzheimer's-related damage. A recent study published in the *Archives of Neurology* suggests that a daily walk or jog could lower the risk of Alzheimer's—or at the very least dull its impact once it has begun. In 2000, Dutch researchers found that inactive men who were genetically prone to Alzheimer's were four times more likely to develop the disease than those who carried the trait but worked out regularly.

In terms of weight loss, exercise can help burn calories. By burning these calories your body uses this energy instead of storing it as fat, but there is also a secondary benefit. Certain forms of exercise affect the metabolism long after you stop doing the actual exercise. For example, you burn calories both during and after strength training because, once you've finished exercising, your body continues to burn calories making and maintaining the muscle tissue. Strength training can actually boost your metabolism by 15%, which can be a huge help in any weight loss strategy.

The list of the exercise benefits is long and getting longer, but I'm not going to spend a lot of time on this because quite frankly you've probably heard most of this a thousand times. Let's move on to something you probably haven't heard.

Why you need to get out of your chair

Most of us wouldn't think of standing around as being "active." But some of the top scientists from around the world involved in sedentary studies would beg to differ. The simple act of standing works our body in a very fundamental way. Standing is actually a basic position for the human body. It's what we were designed to do. On the other hand sitting, the activity that we spend most of our day doing really isn't an activity at all and is actually not what our bodies were designed to do. According to Joan Vernikos PhD, former Director of NASA's Life Sciences Division and Space Medicine Director who worked with astronauts in space, we need to work against gravity to be healthy. "We know gravity pulls down to the center of the earth, and it exerts its maximum effect when we stand up. Standing up often is what matters, not how long you remain standing. Every time you stand up, the body initiates a shift in fluids, volume, and hormones, and causes muscle contractions to occur; and almost every nerve in the body is stimulated. If you stand up 16 times a day for two minutes, the body would read that as 16 stimuli, whereas if you stood once and remained standing for 32 minutes, it would see that as one stimulus."

Why is that so important? Well, we basically have two kinds of muscles. We have "mobilizers," which in the fitness world we call mover muscles, or those muscles we tend to exercise. These are the big muscle groups that do a lot of the heavy lifting that goes on during the day. Then we have "stabilizer" muscles whose job it is to maintain the body's posture. Mover muscles tend to tire quickly and tend to go dormant (little or no electrical activity when not being fully utilized) when not pushing pulling lifting or running. Basically they burn fuel when you're working hard then take a little nap until you need them again. The stabilizer muscles tend to always be awake as long as you're upright. These muscles don't tire very quickly and they are greedy little buggers using lots and lots of energy, as they constantly fight the forces of gravity.

So what's the big difference between sitting and standing, you ask? According to Marc Hamilton, Ph.D., associate professor of biomedical sciences at the University of Missouri, "People need to understand that the qualitative mechanisms of sitting are completely different from walking or exercising…Sitting too much is not the same as exercising too little. They do completely different things to the body."

You might think that just standing around seems every bit as lazy as sitting. Dr. Hamilton knows better. "If you're standing around and puttering, you recruit specialized muscles designed for postural support that never tire," he says. "They're unique in that the nervous system recruits them for low-intensity activity and they're very rich in enzymes." One enzyme, lipoprotein lipase, sucks fat and cholesterol from the blood stream, and burns the fat for energy while shifting the cholesterol from LDL (the bad kind of cholesterol) to HDL (the healthy kind of cholesterol). When you're sitting, the muscles are relaxed, and enzyme activity drops by 90% to 95%, leaving fat to hang out in the bloodstream. After a couple hours of sitting, healthy cholesterol drops by 20%. Amazingly this is just one of the myriad of chemical changes that take place in the body while we sit. Sitting for extended periods of time has a huge cascade of effects on the body—everything from back pain, restricted blood flow, heart disease, diabetes and sitting is also being implicated in an elevated risk of certain types of cancer.

So just how important is getting yourself upright throughout the day? A growing body of evidence says that it could actually extend your life. That's what a new Australian study that looked at death rates over a three-year period had to say. The study concluded that people who spent a lot of time sitting at a desk or in front of a television were more likely to die sooner than those who were only sedentary a few hours a day. The lead author of the study Hidde van der Ploeg and his colleagues at the University of Sydney found that of more than 200,000 adults age 45 and older who reported sitting for at least 11 hours daily were 40 percent more likely to die during the study than those who sat less than 4 hours daily. *40 percent!* The results appear in the Archives of Internal Medicine, March 26, 2012, and reveal that the link between too much time sitting and shortened lives stuck even when they accounted for how much moderate or vigorous exercise people got, as well as their weight and other measures of health.

Another study released in July of 2012 showed that an analysis of five large studies following about 2 million people (not a *small* study at all) in several different countries lead by Peter Katzmarzyk of Louisiana State University's Pennington Biomedical research Center found that the life expectancies of people who said they spent more than three hours a day sitting were a full two years less than people who spent less than three hours sitting daily. Maybe even more surprising was that this was true regardless of whether subjects reported getting the recommended amounts of exercise or not.

Then came the study in the October 2012 edition of The American Journal of Kidney Disease which found that after surveying more than 6,000 adults, the ones that spent the least amount of time in the seated position had the lowest risk for developing chronic kidney disease, regardless of the amount of regular moderate to vigorous sustained exercise they got.

Even more convincing research on the subject comes from The Journal Diabetologia released October 14th 2012, which found a link between sedentary behavior and health risk. The British researchers analyzed the data from 18 studies that had more than 793,000 participants. What they discovered was that people who sat for long periods of time over the course of the day had a two-fold increased risk of diabetes, heart disease and premature death. Again exercise had little or no effect.

A study released in November 2012 showed that people who sat for extended periods during the day accumulated a particularly unhealthy form of fat around the heart. What's more, the fat stayed in place even when people undertook regular exercise. CT scans of more than 500 older Americans found that excess time spent sitting "was significantly related to pericardial fat around your heart," said study lead author Britta Larsen, a postdoctoral researcher in the department of cardiovascular epidemiology at the University of California, San Diego. This particular study looked at data on 504 Californian adults, whose average age was 65. Larsen's team examined CT scan data that showed how much of certain types of body fat were deposited in each participant's body. "We looked at subcutaneous fat, which is stuff on the outside [for example, a "pot belly"]; then visceral fat, which is around your organs; intramuscular fat, which is actually in your muscles; intrathoracic [chest cavity] fat; and pericardial fat, which is around your heart," Larsen said. The people involved in the study were also asked about how much time per week they spent sitting and how much time they had spent being physically active.

What the researchers found was the more time spent sitting, the bigger the area of fat deposited around a person's heart. Larsen explained that pericardial fat "is strongly related to cardiovascular disease. It gets in the way of heart function, it clogs up your arteries -- you don't want it there."

If you would like to read more research on this subject you can read my book Is Your Chair Killing You?, Joan Vernikos' book Sitting Kills Moving Heals, or Dr. James Levine's book Move a

Little Lose a Lot. All three these books are available at Amazon.com.

Beyond just getting out of your chair, another way to workout at work is to do ultra low intensity movements. The pioneer in this research is Dr. James Levine of the Mayo clinic who has devoted more than 20 years of his life to the study of NEAT. NEAT, or non-exercise activity thermogenesis, is a really fancy way of describing the movements that make up your daily life. We're not talking about exercise, just everyday stuff like walking to the bathroom, picking up a stapler, standing up when your boss comes into your cubicle, running the vacuum in the living room, chewing gum, and even picking your nose. It is these everyday movements, not exercise, which made our forefathers "active." In fact, historically speaking, exercise as we know it was an anomaly, not the norm.

What Dr. Levine has discovered in those 20-plus years is that we are doing less NEAT movements and a lot more sitting. The problem is that sitting is one of the most sedentary things you can do and as a society, we do more sitting today than ever before in human history. It hardly seems a coincidence that we are also heavier today than at any other time in human history, which is exactly why we need to concentrate on these low intensity movements. For the office we are going to enhance our ability to do low intensity activities while still concentrating on doing the job at hand, which of course is our work.

The big benefit of these low intensity movements is their ability to burn large quantities of calories. In fact I believe that these low intensity movements are a far more effective way to lose weight than traditional exercise. Their effectiveness hinges on the law of frequency. Exercise has a cumulative effect when it comes to health benefits. In other words 60 minutes of exercise is 60 minutes of exercise whether you do it in 3 minute increments or all in one session. By being more active all day long you're burning little bits of energy over a long period of time and that really adds up. In fact we burn far more energy doing everyday things than we do when we are exercising.

A great analogy for that is fuel efficiency in your car. Does your typical car get better gas mileage while driving on the freeway or in city traffic? Typically highway driving is far more fuel efficient (you burns less gas) than city driving. The start stop, speed up, slow down burns a lot of energy and just isn't very efficient. But going at a steady pace makes fuel consumption go down, improving efficiency. The same is true of your body, but with your body we want to burn more energy so doing more start-stop-speed-up-slow-down helps us burn more calories. Exercise tends to be more like highway driving—moderate to high intensity work done at a steady pace that allows your body to adapt to that activity and become efficient at using its energy. On top of that most of us can only maintain that level of exertion for so long either because of time constraints or because we get tired. By doing it intermittently over the day we will tend to do more and burn more energy. The problem is most of us don't do much at work but sit in our chairs hunched over the computer for hours on end which just happens to be one of the most sedentary things you can do. Bringing short, frequent bursts of movement to your day can be a big help in shedding those unwanted pounds.

Still don't believe me? Here are some real life numbers for you: A person who is chair-bound will burn roughly 300 calories above his or her Basal Metabolic Rate (BMR), or the amount of calories your body burns just staying alive. A person who sits at a desk for most of the day, but gets up for lunch and a few water and restroom breaks, will burn roughly 700 calories over his or her BMR. A person who spends the majority of the day at a desk but manages to move around moderately (goes to the copier down the hall, makes several trips to the file room, walks to the water cooler) will burn 1000 calories over his or her BMR. The person whose job entails mostly standing or is very active will burn 1400 calories over his or her BMR, and the person who has a strenuous job, such as agricultural labor, can burn as much as 2,300 calories over his or her BMR. In order to lose one pound, you have to burn 3500 more calories than you take in. That basically boils down to burning 500 more calories a day than you take in to lose a pound a week, so you can see why being more active during the day makes it easier to lose weight.

A 130 pound woman who runs at a pace of 5 miles per hour (a light jog) will burn 216 calories in 30 minutes. That same woman running at a 9 mile an hour pace (a pretty fast jog) will burn 380 calories. 380 calorie sounds like a lot. But did you know that the difference between simply sitting motionless and standing motionless for the average person is 60 calories an hour? Now I know what you're thinking "Kent, 60 calories isn't anything, heck that's not even a quarter of a Snickers bar." But simply stand for 8 hours (not moving at all) and you burn 480 calories. Now add in some movement to that, just little stuff like walking around, climbing a few stairs, maybe some of the *Office Workout* movements, and you can see the fuel efficiency/inefficiency analogy at work in your life and on your waistline!

On top of the simple calorie burn we get from increased activity, there is also a more complex biochemical process that happens on a cellular level (which is what Marc Hamilton is talking about). This process helps burn sugars and fats that can damage your metabolism, and an efficient, strong, and healthy metabolism keeps you slim and trim. All of this may seem very technical, but what I am basically saying is it is more than just calories in and calories out. Working out at work with low intensity movements has the potential to be a big help in your efforts to drop a few pounds.

More than just losing a few pounds this system also shows potential for being very good for your overall health. A Harvard study that followed more than fifteen hundred women for 30 years to find out what types of physical activity had the most health benefits. They tracked how much exercise what kinds of sports and how active they were. What the study found was the activity that gave the women the most protection against heart disease was walking. Yep, just walking. For the most part it seems that our bodies were designed to do low intensity work all day long and it's beginning to look like we need that near-constant movement to be healthy. The problem is that most of us have days that are filled with almost no movement as we sit at our desks in front of our computers, then we head home to sit on the couch in front of our television.

5
Helping Your Boss See the Light

So how do you get your company or boss to get on board with this whole *Office Workout* thing? Speak to them in a language they can understand...speak to them in the language of money! You can download this chapter as a white paper PDF titled “How to Save Big Money by Letting Your Employees Get Moving at Work” at the home page of my website (www.mylifefitness.com, click on "Workout at Work Boss Guide") and print it or email it to them. This chapter is loaded with research, facts and statistics, and if that's not your thing, you might want to move on to chapter 5.

A recent study in Australia found that metabolic diseases cost Australian businesses 4 billion dollars a year. I'd be willing to bet the number is a lot bigger than that here in the good old U.S.A. Now businesses here in America have certainly recognized the fact that unhealthy workers can negatively affect the bottom line but most business owners and the people responsible for keeping businesses thriving know that keeping their employees healthy is vital to keeping their business healthy. After all I think it's pretty safe to say that employees who are healthy tend to be more vibrant, creative and productive than those who are sick or in constant pain. Let's face it, employees are the life blood of any business and the company needs them at work every business day doing what (hopefully) they do best, manufacturing product, giving great customer service, coming up with new ideas and systems, selling, creating code or whatever it is those employees do to keep the business up, running and profitable. People who are sick or in pain aren't doing that to the best of their ability and people who aren't at work aren't doing it at all.

But the prevailing wisdom in business has been that employers have very little control over the health of their workers. Many businesses have made token efforts like exercise incentive programs and health fairs that brought in nutritionists, personal trainers and health insurance carriers once a year during open enrollment to encourage living a more healthy lifestyle. A few brave businesses (with deep pockets) even went as far as to build company gyms or exercise studios for employees to use before or after work and put into place employee lunch programs with healthy food choices often subsidized by the company to keep it affordable for the rank and file workers. The average manager believed that most of the heavy lifting when it came to the health of your employees was done outside of working hours when the employer had little or no control over what people did during their free time. Free time outside of the proverbial 9 to 5 workday was where people got healthy or got out of shape and little could be done about it by the company. This could be pretty frustrating considering the amount of money unhealthy and injured workers cost businesses both big and small each year. But most CEOs, upper-level managers and business owners threw up their hands and said "Oh well, what can I do about it?" and chalked it up to the price of doing business.

However, a growing body of research is pointing to the fact that the prevailing wisdom is dead wrong and that what employees do (and don't do) at work has a profound impact on their health, creativity *and* productivity. And just as important, this is impacting the businesses bottom line—and not in a good way. Even more surprising is that the efforts of the employees outside of work at the gym or exercise studio may not be enough to overcome the damage that 8 or more hours each day, five or more days a week of sitting behind a desk hunched over a computer does to the body. Unfortunately this is the plight of many American office workers because "productivity experts" created office spaces that for the most part chained workers to their desks, everything from printers to staplers were posted within easy reach of every worker and email insured that they never needed to leave there chair to do anything in the office.

Sedentary Studies research has begun to reveal that our modern work environment is quite literally killing our workforce and with it our businesses. So your workplace is a pretty typical modern day workplace. There are offices and cubicles, desks, chairs, computers and telephones; all of the stuff you would expect to see at an ordinary American office. The people who work at your office are pretty typical too. They spend most of their day at their desk working on the computer or talking on the phone. Some of them are a little over weight (ok, *most* of them are a little over weight) and some of them have some health issues such as diabetes, obesity, heart disease and back problems which are pretty common in the U.S today. Most likely these people are hard workers that spend long hours at the job. Again, there's nothing uncommon there. So what's all the fuss about? Keeping this typical office running is expensive! Let's look at a little case study:

A small rural county in Wisconsin with 600 employees had a $9 million annual budget in 2012. In 2011 more than $ 1.3 million of that budget was spent on healthcare costs for their employees. That's a whopping 14.5percent of their total budget went for employee healthcare costs alone! That doesn't include the costs of lost productivity from sick days or what the employees had to pay out of pocket. Even worse, that number is expected to rise by 9% in 2013.

So clearly reigning in health care costs could go a long way towards improving a business' bottom line. But how exactly do you reign in those costs? Well one way is to have fewer employees need healthcare by preventing them from getting sick—and some of the most expensive and prevalent diseases today are actually pretty preventable. These diseases are known as metabolic diseases and include diabetes, heart disease and obesity. We also know that the chances of getting other diseases like stroke, kidney disease some forms of cancer and even back pain can be diminished through preventative measures. So reining in your health care costs could go a long way towards improving your bottom line.

So let's start by talking about just how much money these illnesses are really costing you and your business.

Cost of Diabetes to Employers

From the Centers for Disease Control:

Diabetes does affect corporate America and its bottom line.

• In 2007, direct and indirect costs of diabetes total nearly $174 billion a year.

• People with diagnosed diabetes, on average have medical expenditures that are 2.3 times higher than what the expenditures would be in the absence of diabetes.

• In 2007, indirect costs include increased absenteeism ($2.6 billion) and reduced productivity while at work ($20.0 billion for the employed population, reduced productivity for those not in the labor force ($0.8 billion), unemployment from disease- related disability ($7.9 billion) and lost productive capacity due to early mortality ($26.9 billion).

• Diabetes accounts for 15 million work days absent, 120 million work days with reduced performance, 107 million work days lost due to unemployment disability attributed to diabetes.

• People with diabetes have a health related absenteeism rate that is 0.8% higher than people without diabetes.

• The population with the highest per capita productivity loss from absenteeism is males age 45-53.

The cost of health care for people with diabetes is 230 percent more expensive than for people without diabetes according to the American Diabetes Association. This statistic has been confirmed by a recent report from United Healthcare, which compiled data from 10 million members and found that the average annual health care costs in 2009 for a person with known diabetes were about $11,700 compared with about $4,400 for the non-diabetic public – 260 percent more expensive. In fact, by the end of this decade it is estimated that medical care for pre diabetes and diabetes will account for ten percent of the total healthcare spending in the U.S. Employers will bare a significant portion of this financial burden.

In fact diabetes has been identified as the 3rd most costly physical health condition for employers.

Direct medical, disability and absenteeism costs determined for a pool of 375,000 employees from 6 large corporations revealed:

• Annual diabetes-related costs totaled $104 per employee, even though only 4.8% actually had diabetes

• Each employee with diabetes cost an average of $21,000 a year

The cost of treating diabetes and its complications is a heavy burden on employee health plans. More than 10% of all U.S. healthcare expenditures in 2002 went to treat the disease and its associated complications. By 2050, the annual cost will top $132-billion, the bulk of that for treating complications. In a just-released study of diabetes trends, researchers predict that the increasingly complex and costly diabetes treatments will have a significant impact on the provision of health care to those patients.

Diabetes drug expenditures leaped from $6.7 billion in 2001 to $12.5 billion in 2007 A prime cost driver was the increased use of newer and more costly drugs. The mean price of a diabetes drug prescription has increased from $56 in 2001 to $76 in 2007.

Costs associated with diabetes are weighing heavily on employers and employees alike. United Healthcare claims for uncomplicated diabetes rose from $45 million per year in the 4th quarter of 2005 to $49 million in the 3rd quarter of 2007. Complicated diabetes costs increased from $64 million to $73 million over the same time period.

Employers face an additional, hidden cost from the effects of diabetes. Employees who do not properly care for themselves, take their medications, and get regular professional care cost millions of dollars annually to presenteeism, the situation where an ill employee reports to work but is not able to work to full capacity. Employee effectiveness can be reduced as much as 50% in many presenteeism cases.

Corporate America can help employees manage their diabetes or reduce their risks of developing it.

• With employees spending more than one-third of their days on the job, corporate America is in a unique position to address this health issue.

• It is in the employer's best interest to try to work with their employees who have diabetes or are at risk for the disease to improve productivity and lower health costs as well as help employees stay in good mental and physical health.

• Control the ABCs (A1c, Blood Pressure, Cholesterol)

• **Glucose Control.** In general, every percentage point drop in A1C blood glucose reduces the risk of micro vascular complications (eye, kidney and nerve diseases) by 40%.

• **Blood Pressure Control.** Reduces the risk of cardiovascular disease (heart disease or stroke) by 33% to 50% and the risk of micro vascular complications by approximately 33%.

• **Control of Blood Lipids.** Improved control of cholesterol or blood lipids (e.g., HDL, LDL and triglycerides) can reduce cardiovascular complications by 20% to 50%.

• **Preventive Care Practices for Eyes, Feet and Kidneys.**

-Detecting and treating diabetes eye disease with laser therapy can reduce the development of severe vision loss by an estimated 50% to 60.

-Comprehensive foot care programs can reduce amputation rates by 45% to 85%.

-Detecting and treating early diabetic kidney disease by lowering blood pressure can reduce kidney function decline by 30% to 70%.

-Current data from the American Diabetes Association: shows that people with diabetes that control their disease by keeping their blood sugar down cost employers only $24 a month, compared with the $115 a month for people with diabetes who do not control their blood sugar.

Diabetes prevention is proven, possible, and powerful.

• Studies show that people at high risk for type 2 diabetes can prevent or delay the onset of the disease by losing 5 to 7 percent of their body weight, by eating healthier and getting 30 minutes of physical activity 5 days a week. The key is: small steps that lead to big rewards.

These are just the costs for businesses; when you look at the overall dollars spent on diabetes the numbers are staggering. Diabetes affects nearly 25 million Americans and is the fifth leading cause of death in America, killing more than breast cancer and AIDs combined. According to a report from the Agency for Healthcare Research and Quality, this lifestyle disease is costing Americans $83 billion a year in hospital fees alone, that's 23 % of total hospital spending. According to the 2007 report "Economic Costs of Diabetes in the U.S." the overall cost of diabetes is $174 billion ($116 billion in direct costs like medical expenditures, including drugs, office visits, and hospital costs, and $58 billion in indirect costs such as reduced national productivity). Some other amazing stats:

• One of every five health care dollars is spent caring for someone with diabetes.

• Diabetics have medical expenditures that are 2.3 times higher than other victims of chronic disease.

• Diabetics have more frequent facility stays, more home health visits, and more prescription drug and supply usage.

When you throw in the costs of the hidden diabetes epidemic, that means the 6.3 million people that have the disease but haven't been diagnosed and the 57 million Americans that are considered pre-

diabetic (likely to develop type 2 diabetes within 10 years), that $174 billion figure goes up another $43 billion dollars.
According to the authors of the report "The burden of diabetes is imposed on all sectors of society- higher insurance premiums paid by employees and employers, reduced earnings through productivity loss, and reduced overall quality of life for people with diabetes and their families and friends." Interestingly enough, diet and exercise alone can help prevent or control type 2 diabetes, which accounts for 95% of all cases of diabetes, meaning that many of these economic and human costs could be saved.

Costs of Heart Disease and Stroke to Employers

In 2009, the economic costs of cardiovascular diseases and stroke were estimated at $475.3 billion, including $313.8 billion in direct medical expenses and $161.5 billion in indirect costs ($39.1 in lost productivity due to sickness or disability and $122.4 lost productivity due to premature death)10

According to the health website Web MD, in the U.S., all cardiovascular diseases, including heart conditions, stroke, peripheral artery disease, and high blood pressure combined cost $273 billion each year. In fact, of all the money spent in the U.S. on health care, 17% goes toward treating cardiovascular disease, says Paul A. Heidenreich, MD, a cardiologist at the Veterans Administration Palo Alto Health Care System in Palo Alto, California and Associate Professor of Medicine at Stanford University. Heart conditions such as heart failure, heart attack, and surgical procedures such as bypasses account for nearly $96 billion of that total. That, my friends, is a gigantic load of cash.

Ok, so these numbers are figured on a pretty big scale, but what about the costs per person? A recent study published in *Circulation*, the *Journal of the American Heart Association* estimated that over the course of one person's lifetime, the cost of severe coronary artery disease -- the most common form of heart disease -- is more than $1 million. That includes both direct and indirect costs. Direct costs, like ambulance transportation, diagnostic tests, hospitalization, and possible surgery and a pacemaker or implantable defibrillator can add up quickly. Long-term maintenance of heart disease is also expensive, including medications, testing, and cardiologist appointments. It's harder to grasp the indirect costs of heart disease, but they can be enormous. The biggest are lost productivity and income. Many people might be able to return to work a few months after having a heart attack, but even losing income for a few months can cause grave financial problems. Surveys show that most people would be only 90 days away from bankruptcy if they stopped getting paid. For people with a severe disease, it can be difficult to return to work full time, and some may never be able to return at all. Even worse, those who don't have good health insurance, or insurance at all, can be financially ruined by heart disease seemingly overnight. Apart from the direct costs, the lost wages alone can be crippling.

Some of you might be thinking to yourself that you don't have to worry about the costs of heart disease; you've had your cholesterol checked and your blood-pressure is in a healthy range. But the truth is, even if you don't develop heart disease, it's still costing you. "You're paying for cardiovascular disease whether you have it or not," Heidenreich says. "You're paying for it in your taxes and your health insurance premiums." He estimates that the average person in the U.S. is paying $878 per year for the societal costs of heart disease.

While the cost of care for an individual in the first 30 days following a stroke is only $13,019 in mild cases and $20,346 in severe cases, the lifetime cost of a stroke can add up to approximately $140,048. The bulk of those costs come in the form of chronic care and rehabilitation. Although there have been significant decreases in both the mortality rate (20.7% between 1995 and 2005) and the incidence of strokes (12.8% between 1995 and 2006), this trend is expected to soon reverse itself as the population ages – particularly among ethnic minority groups who are at especially high risk of stroke. Providing there are no changes in treatment, preventative care, or trends of risk factors (i.e. incidence of obesity), the result of this reversal will be an increase in spending on stroke care, from $65.6 billion in 2008 to $2.2 trillion by the year 2050.

Costs of Cancer to Employers

The CDC reports that overall spending on direct care for cancer totaled $74 billion in 2004. While there are no reliable cost projections for cancer, recent years have seen an exponential increase in the cost of cancer drugs, as illustrated in the 2006 *New York Times* article titled "A Cancer Drug's Big Price Rise is Cause for Concern." Cancer treatment is especially prone to spending an exorbitant amount of money on a marginal benefit, with some treatments, such as Avastin – used for metastatic breast, colon, and non-small cell lung cancer – costing over $90,000 for a 1.5-month increase in predicted survival time, or $2,000 per day.

According to the same CDC report, Medicare spent $7.3 billion dollars that year (about ten % of overall cancer spending) on inpatient cancer care, and this total does not even include most chemotherapy, which is administered as an outpatient service and is covered under Part B. Medicare spending on Part B drugs in 2004 totaled $10.87 billion, representing a steady 25% annual increase from the $2.76 billion spent in 1997. Given that the incidence of cancer in people above age 65 is nearly 10 times that of people under 65, as the population ages, Medicare is bound to pay a large and growing portion of the nation's overall spending on cancer treatments. When you consider that chronic diseases account for such a great proportion of Medicare's overall spending, any increases in chronic care spending will directly affect Medicare. This directly affects all Americans because we all contribute to Medicare.

Costs of Obesity to Employers

The dollar figures for the cost of obesity are high because being obese often leads to having one or more of the other lifestyle diseases. The CDC roughly defines obesity as being 30 pounds over your ideal weight. According to a report published in the online edition of *Health Affairs,* in the United States $147 billion per year is spent on direct medical expenses for obesity, which is just over 9% of all medical spending. Furthermore, obesity is the number two cause of preventable death in the United States. To say that obesity has reached epidemic proportions in the U.S. is actually a bit of an understatement. The statistics are mind-numbing. The Get America Fit Foundation cites the following statistics:

• 58 million Americans are overweight
• 40 million are obese
• 3 million are morbidly obese
• 8 out of 10 over the age of 25 are overweight
• 80% of all type 2 diabetes is related to obesity
• 70% of cardiovascular disease is related to obesity
• Type 2 diabetes costs $63.14 billion per year
• Heart disease costs $6.9 billion per year
• Work days lost due to obesity-related issues cost $39.3 million per year
• Physician office visits cost $62.7 million per year
• Restricted activity days cost $29.9 million per year

The increasing costs of being overweight or obese to individuals, businesses and to society as a whole are astounding. According to a report sponsored by the United Health Foundation and the American Public Health Association, the cost of medical-related expenses from obesity in 2018 could soar to over $344 billion a year. The calculations are based on the projections that, if obesity continues to rise at the current rate, 43% of American adults may be obese. Honestly there are loads more statistics that I could beat you over the head with, but after a while my eyes start to roll back in my head and my teeth hurt.

So let's move on to some happy news. You can save yourself a whole lot of money and even more grief and heartache by doing a few simple things. First, eat a healthy, well-balanced diet, including lots of fruits and vegetables. Personally, I believe in a real food diet that is heavily influenced by the Mediterranean diet, but there are thousands of nutrition books out there so you can find the one that works for you. Next, you need to simply (and I mean SIMPLY) add more frequent and consistent movement to your predominantly sedentary routine over the course of your day to keep these lifestyle diseases at bay.

If you are currently getting 30 to 60 minutes of moderate cardiopulmonary exercise (walking briskly is good enough) 4 to 6 days a week, that's great, but stay with me here, because we're about to go into why it may not be enough.

Costs of Back Pain to Employers

According to a study in the Journal of the American Medical Association (JAMA), In 2005 Americans spent $85.9 billion looking for relief from back and neck pain through surgery, doctor's visits, X-rays, MRI scans and medications, up from $52.1 billion in 1997, That money hasn't helped reduce the number of sufferers; in 2005, 15 percent of U.S. adults reported back problems—up from 12 percent in 1997.

Not only are more people seeking treatment for back pain, but the price of treatment per person is also up. In the JAMA study, researchers at the University of Washington and Oregon Health & Science University compared national data from 3,179 adult patients who reported spine problems in 1997 to 3,187 who reported them in 2005—and found that inflation-adjusted annual medical costs increased from $4,695 per person to $6,096. Those numbers are up significantly in the year 2012.

According to the American Academy of Pain Medicine back pain American businesses:

• Back pain (BP) in workers 40 to 65 years of age costs employers an estimated $7.4 billion/year.

• 71.6% of this cost is due to workers with BP exacerbations

• 42.6% of all workers reported BP exacerbations, even though BP prevalence is associated with demographic factors.

• The 2-week prevalence of BP was 15.1%; with 42% of workers with back pain (BP) experienced pain exacerbations

• Workers with exacerbations reported more days with BP than those without exacerbations.

• Workers with exacerbations were significantly more likely than those without such exacerbations to report activity limitation and BP-related lost productive time.

Workers with BP exacerbations account for a disproportionate share of the cost of BP-related lost productive time. Remember that back pain is the number 2 reason for sick calls in America only behind the common cold and flu.

Now I've had business owners say to me, "Kent, I'm a small business owner and I don't have health insurance for my workers so I don't have all those expenses" My answer to them is "you're swimming in a large river in Egypt my friend because you are most definitely in de-Nile"...Okay, that's a bad joke. But if your employees don't have health insurance they probably are putting off going to the doctor, which means that their condition is getting worse. They don't feel good and aren't being as productive as they could be. When they finally do see a doctor their condition will be far worse and they will have to be treated in a far more aggressive manner and will probably have to stay out of work for several days or maybe even several weeks….which of course costs you money. Maybe they get so sick that they have to go on disability or quit. Now you have to replace them, which means you have to find someone, which takes time and money, and then train them. You see where I'm going with this: the bottom line is if you don't offer health insurance to your people you had better be far more invested in preventative steps for your work force to keep them healthy, happy and- more importantly for your business-at work and doing their jobs.

Want to see just how big a savings we're talking about? That small rural county in Wisconsin with 600 employees has a $9 million annual budget. Last year more than $ 1.3 million of that budget was spent on healthcare costs for their employees. The county's employee wellness program participation rate was less than 5%, which is pretty average. This means that the county provided the employees with after work classes and smoking cessations programs as well as other health and wellness benefits as a part of their wellness program. But less than 5% of the employees took advantage of those programs.

The Department of Health and Human Performance at East Carolina University has created an inactivity calculator that estimates a business or government's potential savings if they could get more inactive people to become active (if you would like to know how the calculator was created and what parameters it uses you can check it out at http://www.ecu.edu/picostcalc/).

According to the calculator this rural Wisconsin county could have saved $72,126 dollars a year by simply getting 5 percent more of their workforce involved in their wellness program. They could save over $500,000 dollars a year if they could just get 50% of their employees involved in the wellness program. So, getting people to do an office workout is a fiscally sound proposition, especially if it only takes a few minutes every hour. Wave half a million dollars in the face of even the most old school employer and I guarantee you'll get their attention.

The following is data from the Wellness Councils of America and will give you an idea of just how much money can be saved by improving the health of a company's employees. Keep in mind these are the dollar figures from a traditional wellness program, these numbers could be considerably larger if a company was to get a significant number of their employees to do the *Office Workout* program at their desk daily.

From the Wellness Councils of America website:

Today, more than 81% of America's businesses with 50 or more employees have some form of health promotion program the most popular being exercise, stop-smoking classes, back care programs, and stress management. Most employers offer wellness programs simply because they think the benefit is worth the cost. Yet business leaders continue to ask themselves how to control huge annual increases in health insurance premiums and health care costs.

For many companies, medical costs can consume half of corporate profits or more. Some employers look to cost sharing, cost shifting, managed care plans, risk rating, and cash-based rebates or incentives. But these methods merely shift costs. Only worksite health promotion stands out as the long-term answer for keeping employees well in the first place.

Worksite wellness is health care reform that works. Results from America's finest companies, summarized here, are reason enough to think about an investment in your most important asset--your employees and the impact this investment can have on your bottom line.

Providence Everett Medical Center, a member of the Wellness Councils of America, in Everett, Washington, saved an estimated 3 million or a cost-benefit ratio of 1 to 3.8 over 9 years of an outcomes-based employee health benefit program called *The Wellness Challenge®*. By offering financial incentives ($250 - $325) to employees who meet specific organizational and employee health initiatives the program continues to meet cost containment expectations in the area of healthcare use, sick time, injuries, while improving health habits and self-care practices. During the first 4 years of the program there was a 28% average reduction in healthcare utilization compared to nine other Providence hospitals that were used as a control group.

Du Pont saw that each dollar invested in workplace health promotion yielded $1.42 over two years in lower absenteeism costs at Du Pont Co. (Well Workplace Gold in Delaware). Absences from illness unrelated to the job among 45,000 blue-collar workers dropped 14% at 41 industrial sites where the health promotion program was offered, compared with a 5.8% decline at 19 sites where it was not.

The Travelers Corporation claims a $3.40 return for every dollar invested in health promotion, yielding total corporate savings of $146 million in benefits costs. Sick leave was reduced 19% during the four-year study. In addition to improving the overall health of 36,000 employees and retirees by reducing poor health habits and increasing good ones, The Travelers realized cost savings by decreasing the number of unnecessary visits to a doctor and emergency rooms. In a similar but smaller study, members of a Travelers fitness center were absent from work significantly fewer days than nonmembers.

The Stay Alive & Well program at Reynolds Electrical & Engineering Company, based in Las Vegas, cost $76.24 per employee during the two years it has been in operation. Over half of the 1,600 employees participated (with up to 80% participation rates in the intervention program). Participants significantly lowered cholesterol levels, blood pressure, and weight and experienced 21% lower lifestyle-related claim costs than non-participant. Resulting savings: $127.89 per participant with a benefit to cost ratio of 1.68 to 1.

Superior Coffee and Foods, a Bensenville-Illinois-based subsidiary of Sara Lee Corporation, attributes impressive results to the success of the company's comprehensive wellness program. Superior showed 22% fewer admissions to a hospital, 29% shorter hospital stays, and 42% lower expenses per admission when comparing costs for this division's 1,200 employees with costs for other divisions. Long-term disability costs were down by 40%. Superior Coffee and Foods has earned WELCOA's Well Workplace Gold award.

With medical costs per employee at $6,000, nearly twice the national average, Union Pacific Railroad introduced the concept of personal health management to its 28,000 employees, mostly union and blue collar, in 19 Western and Southern states. Beginning with a modest medical self-care initiative at an annual cost of $50 per person, the program achieved a net savings of

$1.26 million. In addition, a voluntary program to help employees lower health risks projected a cost-benefit ratio of 1 to 1.57 after one year. Employees in a treatment group lowered their risk of high blood pressure (45%) and high cholesterol (34%); others moved out of the at-risk range for weight problems (30%); and 21% stopped smoking.

Average medical costs of high-risk Steelcase employees--those whose lifestyles include two to four health risks such as smoking, little exercise, overweight--are 75% higher than those of low-risk employees. But high-risk employees at this Grand Rapids, Michigan-furniture manufacturing company who improved their health habits through the company's health promotion program and became low risk cut their average medical claims in half thus lowering their medical insurance costs by an average of $618 per year. If all high-risk employees (20% of the total employee population) in one location changed their lifestyles to become low risk, the projected savings could total $20 million over three years.

Employees at Berk-Tec, a small manufacturing company in Lancaster County Pennsylvania, learned self-care techniques and lowered their company's health care costs in one year. By using a self-care guide, the 938 employees and their family members made smart medical decisions and saved $21.67 per employee and dependent--a nearly 18% reduction in costs. By combining reductions in doctor visits and emergency room use, the company saved $39.06 per employee a 24.3% decrease in costs over the previous year.

A medical claims-based study of 72,000 people insured through 285 Wisconsin school districts found a lower demand for medical services among those with access to disease prevention and self-care programs. Reductions in medical services resulted in savings for the Wisconsin Education Insurance Group of as much as $4.75 for each $1 spent, and higher savings were found in the group receiving access to a 24-hour phone-based nurse advice line, a self-care reference book, and health education materials.

CIGNA's Healthy Babies Prenatal Program delivered an average savings of $5,000 per birth by providing expectant mothers with educational materials and rewarding early and regular prenatal care. And 80% of participants had normal births without complications compared with 50% for non-participant. CIGNA is a member of the Wellness Councils of America.

With savings estimated to be as high as $8 million, the California Public Employees' Retirement System sent its 55,000 retirees a health risk appraisal followed, in some cases, with individualized reports and letters and self-care materials to encourage change and help reduce health risks among retirees and at the same time reduce the health care claim costs. In another study, Bank of America retirees in California who chose the full health promotion and demand reduction program showed a decrease in total direct and indirect costs of 11% compared with an increase of 6.3% for those who completed only a simple health questionnaire.

With lower health care claims, medical costs decreased 16% for employees in the City of Mesa (Arizona) who participated in the comprehensive health promotion program. The city realized a return of $3.60 for every dollar invested in the health of city employees.

To prevent back injuries among its employees, a county in California targeted white- and blue-collar workers, offered classes and fitness training. As a result, there was a significant increase in employee morale, reduced worker's comp claims, medical costs and sick days related to back injuries producing a net cost-benefit ratio of 1 to 1.79.

References

Wisconsin Education Insurance Group: Internal study conducted by the OPTUM division of United Healthcare Corporation, 1995.

Bank of America: Two-year results of a randomized controlled trial of a health promotion program in a retiree population: The Bank of America study. James F. Fries, D.A. Bloch, Harry Harrington, Nancy Richardson, Robert Beck. American Journal of Medicine, 1993, vol. 94, pp. 455-462.

Berk-Tec: The effect of a medical self-care program on health care utilization. Don R. Powell, Stephanie L. Sharp, Shelley Farnell, P. Timothy Smith. 1996. In press.

California County: A cost-benefit analysis of a California county's back injury prevention program. L. Shi. Public Health Reports, 1993, vol. 108, no. 2, pp. 204-211.

California Public Employees' Retirement System: Randomized controlled trial of cost reductions from a health education program: The California Public Employees' Retirement System (PERS) Study. James F. Fries, Harry Harrington, Robert Edwards, Louis A. Kent, Nancy Richardson. American Journal of Health Promotion, vol. 8, no. 3, pp. 216-223.

CIGNA: CIGNA Healthy Babies program is delivering healthier babies. National Underwriter, Sept. 12, 1994. Stewart Beltz, Director of CIGNA Employee Health Management, press release.

City of Mesa: Influence of a mobile worksite health promotion program on health care costs. S.G. Aldana, B.H. Jacobson, C.J. Harris, P.L. Kelley, W.J. Stone. American Journal of Preventive Medicine, 1994, vol. 9, no. 6, pp. 378-382.

Du Pont: The effects of workplace health promotion on absenteeism and employment costs in a large industrial population. Robert L. Bertera. American Journal of Public Health, September 1990, vol. 80, no. 9, pp. 1101-1105.

Providence General Hospital: Controlled trial of a financial incentive program as a component of a hospital-based worksite health promotion program. Larry Chapman. 1996. In publication. Providence General Medical Center press release, June 19, 1995.

Reynolds Electrical & Engineering Co.: Anthem Health Systems, Inc., Indianapolis, Ind. Staying alive and well at Reynolds Electrical & Engineering Co., Inc., 1993.

Steelcase: Corporate medical claim cost distributions and factors associated with high-cost status. Louis Tze-chingYen, Dee W. Edington, Pamela Witting. Journal of Occupational Medicine, May 1994, vol. 36, no. 5, pp. 505-515.
Superior Coffee and Foods: Speech by Lee Ahsmann, Vice President of Human Resources, at Well Workplace awards dinner, Worksite Wellness Council of Illinois, 1994.
The Travelers: A benefit-to-cost analysis of a worksite health promotion program. Thomas Golaszewski, David Snow, Wendy Lynch, Louis Yen, Debra Solomita. Journal of Occupational Medicine, December 1992, vol. 34, no. 12, pp. 1164-1172. Impact of a facility-based corporate fitness program on the number of absences from work due to illness. Wendy Lynch, Thomas Golaszewski, Andrew Clearie, David Snow, Donald Vickery. Journal of Occupational Medicine, 1990, vol. 32, no. 1, pp. 9-12.
Union Pacific Railroad: Office of the Medical Director, Union Pacific Railroad, Omaha, Neb. Well Workplace Gold award-winning application, 1996. C. Everett Koop Award winner, 1995. U.S. Department of Health and Human Services, National Survey of Worksite Health Promotion Activities (Office of Disease Prevention and Health Promotion), 1992. Obtain the Summary Report from the National Health Information Center, PO Box 1133, Washington, DC 20013-1133.

6
Getting Movement into Your Daily Work Life

Ultra Low-Intensity Cardio

Okay, technically I don't think what I'm about to talk about can actually qualify as "cardio" in the fitness sense of that word, but for lack of a better term I'm going refer to being more active over the course of the work day as "ultra low intensity cardio." In the workplace it's easy to get caught up in what you're doing and find yourself sitting in the exact same position for hours on end. But we know that this is the recipe for disaster or at least a road that leads to ill health, expensive medical bills and lots of time away from work. So how do you keep this from happening? There are some simple things you can do to keep yourself moving for most of the day and staying productive at work. Some of these things will require special tools. I understand that some of these things may not be a viable option for you in your work situation, (that doesn't mean that you can't do them in your home to keep you more active during your off hours) but I would like to provide you with as many tools and options as possible to help you be healthier and more successful.

The first step in this process is to re-think how you have your office set up. Most of us have our desk and office set up so everything is pretty handy. The stapler is in easy reach, the file cabinet is close enough that you don't have to get out of your chair to get those files. The printer is right there on your desktop. It's all very convenient. But convenience isn't necessarily a good thing. The more we get up and move the healthier and happier we're going to be because all that activity is going to increase your metabolism, engage both stabilizer and mover muscles, burn fat and sugars in the bloodstream and pump up blood flow to the brain. By arranging your work station in such a way that you are forced to be more active, changing your habits will become more a matter of necessity than conscious, effortful change. At the office, moving things you use on a regular basis, like staplers, calculators and paper clips to places that force you to get out of your seat to get them is an easy way to increase your activity. Putting file cabinets and the printer on the other side of the room is also helpful. So is switching from a large water bottle you keep on your desk to a small cup that you have to fill at the water cooler across the office when you get thirsty. Spend a few minutes looking at your workspace and do some rearranging that will help you get more movement into your day and a little less sitting. And remember, decrease your fuel efficiency; every little bit helps.

Here's a list of things you can do at the office to be more active.

- Park in the furthest parking space from your destination
- Place regularly used items in an area where you will have to get up to get them
- Always stand and pace when on the phone
- Fidget when sitting for more than twenty minutes (shake your legs, strum your fingers, twirl a pencil or pen)
- Create a stand up desk by placing a wide, sturdy cardboard box on top of your desk and place the keyboard and mouse on it. Use it every half hour.
- Have walking meetings with fellow workers
- Chew sugarless gum
- Drink small cups of water from the water cooler across the office so you'll have to make frequent trips

- Use the bathroom that is furthest from your desk
- Take the stairs instead of the elevator
- If your destination is less than a mile away, walk or ride your bike
- Make every coffee break a walking break
- Stand up and walk around the office every thirty minutes
- Deliver documents and messages to coworkers at their desk instead of calling or emailing
- Leave your lunch in the car or someplace you have to walk to get to it

Movement Motivators

An inexpensive tool that can help you gauge whether or not you're being successful in your effort to be more active is a pedometer. Pedometers come in many different forms and price ranges. Keep in mind that you want a pedometer that is fairly accurate and has the ability to do more than just count the number of steps you take each day. What we're looking for is more overall activity during the day not just how many steps you took. Just going from the seated position to a standing position has health benefits. You can get an inexpensive clip-on pedometer or use one of the many smart phone apps. Personally my favorite pedometer is the Fitbit. The reason I love the Fitbit is that it measures overall activity (it even does it while you sleep allowing you to see how restless you are at night) It also has the ability to sync to your smart phone or computer showing your daily activity in graphs or reports. This product sector is exploding with all kinds of new options too, like smart watches and phone apps. So find the one that works best for you.

Using an exercise ball instead of an office chair is a good start for working out at work. Sitting on the ball forces you to engage many more muscle groups than a traditional office chair and can be used to enhance the workout as you do strength training at your desk. By simply lifting a foot off the floor you effectively work your core, which isn't the case with that bad old office chair. You will notice that in this book series I use the ball extensively in the exercises, so having one is a must.

The exercises in this book are all done with exercise bands or rubber tubing (also known as resistance bands) and hand weights. Bands or tubing are a great option for the office because they store easily, don't weigh anything if you want to schlep them back and forth from home to office, and unlike hand weights they allow a lot of flexibility (they are rubber after all) in how they can be used. Resistance bands come in varying thicknesses, which increases the difficulty of getting them to stretch. Usually they are color coded and come in extra light, light, medium, heavy and extra heavy resistance. You should choose the correct resistance for your fitness level and the muscle group you are working (stronger muscles, higher resistance) which is why you should have several bands in your desk. There are two types of resistance bands: thin rubber bands (that look like bandages made of rubber) and rubber tubing with built-in handles. Personally I prefer tubing. Tubing is more resilient and holds up to heavier use (most of the damage to all forms of resistance bands happens in storage and the office tends to have lots of sharp objects in the same places where you might need to store your equipment) and tubing has a lot of great accessories like handles and door attachments. I especially like the braided tubing for the office, as it lessens the likelihood of the dreaded band break which can be dangerous, painful, loud and embarrassing. When selecting hand weights you should get a weight that challenges you. Each of the exercises in this book are done for very specific amounts of time, you should choose a weight that at the end of the 30 – 60 seconds you are doing the exercise for your muscles feel fatigued.

A good low intensity cardio option is an under-desk pedal machine. These machines are simple and effective, but best of all they are inexpensive! Starting at $30.00 and going up to the low

$100.00 range, these little babies store easily and no one even needs to know they're there under your desk. The calorie burn isn't huge but it's certainly better than just sitting in your chair doing nothing. These puppies can keep you moving all day long even if you can't ever get out of your chair. You can also put them on top of the desk and use your hands to move the pedals, which help you work the upper body. The other great thing about these units is their complete portability. You can take them to the office then grab them as you head home to use in front of the TV.

I think the most valuable tool in the office for good health and weight loss is the stand up desk. While I don't recommend standing all day long (there are some studies that show standing all day increases the risk of varicose veins) standing for 30 minutes and sitting 20 minutes keeps me energized without the tired feet and legs I sometimes get with standing alone. And the health, weight loss, and improved energy benefits are outstanding. Most stand-up desks are desks that are taller than traditional desks and therefore are meant to be used in the standing position. Stand-up desks are not a new phenomenon. In fact, author Ernest Hemingway was said to have used a stand-up desk, as was Secretary of Defense Donald Rumsfeld. Standing desks take a little getting used to, but most people rave about their standing desks after the adjustment period. Mostly you hear about weight loss, disappearing back pain, and increasing energy levels.

My favorite stand up desk is made by Ergotron. The reason I like it is that it's not a conventional stand up desk. It's actually is a combo sit-stand desk that effortlessly moves from a sitting to a standing position whenever you want. The desk I use is customized with accessories to fit individual users' needs and workflow. It has effortless height adjustment that is instantaneous and tool-free, so you can do it while you work! The large sit stand desk runs about $900.00.

Ergotron also offers a WorkFit Station that attaches to your current desk and adjust to your height as you sit or stand. Usually these include an adjustable arm that allows you to move the keyboard and the monitor out of the way when you don't need them. These attachable work stations also give you the flexibility to move from sitting to standing in just seconds, and best of all is the price! While a sit-stand desk can cost around $900, attachable work stations go for around just $495. The other thing I like about the attachable work station is it gives me a nice sturdy platform for attaching my exercise bands and the adjustable height means I can work my muscles from different angles. I have also seen several money-saving designs, such as putting desks up on boxes, and placing monitors and keyboards on flat boards resting on full cases of canned soft drinks, though getting the ergonomics just right can be challenging. Don't be afraid to be creative; this is one of those cases where a little imagination can get you a healthier workspace for very little money.

If you're a cyclist, then the FitDesk is for you. It is designed for people who love to bike but is perfect for the office. I really like the FitDesk stationary bike desk because using it involves activating a large number of the big muscle groups and the smaller postural muscle groups, so the calorie burn is significant. It also has the advantage of being really safe, even for those with very little body awareness (that's a polite term for people like my wife, which is to say *a little klutzy*). This is the grown up version of the pedal machine. They are safe because falling off the bike is far less likely to occur if you get distracted by a call or email and forget to move your feet (which has been known to happen on treadmill desks).What makes this different from an ordinary stationary bike are its low-intensity setting which won't leave you sweaty at the office and its ability to easily and securely hold your lap top computer and a bottle of water. The other thing that makes it both office and home friendly is its ability to fold up and be put away into a relatively small space.

Now for those of you with an unlimited budget and space as well as a boss who is very progressive (if you're the boss and you get this for your employees I take my hat off to you) A treadmill desk is the Rolls Royce of weight-loss/health office furniture from a calorie-burning and postural-muscle-engaging standpoint—it's also the most expensive option. These desks combine exactly what our body was created to do, walking, with the ease of use that a traditional desk offers. Heck, several models even actually incorporate cup holders in the design! The walking pace can be controlled so that you don't feel overwhelmed or get sweaty. The work space can be raised or lowered for ultimate comfort and the potential daily calorie burn is huge. The learning curve for most people is about 3 hours, but after that, the term I've heard most often used to describe the experience is "addictive." The secret seems to be to find the perfect speed for you. Too slow and you can't find a rhythm. Too fast and you'll feel like you're going to fall off while you do your basic daily tasks. But once you find your sweet spot, it's like nirvana. In addition to the physical benefits, most researchers noted better brain function and an increase in alertness and focus throughout the day. Personally, I know that I think more clearly and get more done when I'm walking. In fact, I tend to do my best work while on the move, so the walking desk fits me to a tee. If you're interested in walking and working at the same time you have a couple of different options. If you don't currently have a treadmill, one option is to buy a treadmill that has a desk integrated or attached to it. Traditional treadmills and their motors aren't really designed for day in and day out use at low speeds, so if you plan to use this equipment daily, then a complete system may be a wiser purchase.

However, if you already own a treadmill you can always just buy a desk for it, like the TrekDesk. This type of product is specifically designed to simply fit over the treadmill you already own. I accomplished a similar setup myself with some power tools and a little elbow grease (though in all fairness, mine is pretty ghetto-looking and doesn't have anywhere near the work surface area or cool cup holders). In the office I personally think that the walking desk is best suited for the group meeting setting. Putting four or five of these in a conference room and doing walking meetings is innovative and really helps keep people engaged and alert during meetings. I have it on good authority that the Facebook corporate campus in Menlo Park, California is a virtual wonderland of workplace activity equipment that includes treadmill desks and standing desks, among other workplace productivity-enhancers. Other forward-thinking companies such as Apple, 3M, and GE have recognized the bottom-line benefits of movement in the workplace and actively encourage their employees to work out at work. You have to ask your boss, what CEO or manager wouldn't want to be mentioned in the same breath as Steve Jobs or Mark Zuckerberg? Especially when all they'd have to do to achieve that lofty brotherhood is to say yes to your request to do *The Office Workout!*

In the next part of the book I am going to give you 75 exercises that can be done at your desk. I've created a wide variety of exercises, some of which require simple fitness tools. As you do these exercises, it will be obvious that you are doing a very short micro-workout. But first, here is a bonus chapter with 10 exercises you can do *in your chair* that will improve your health.

7
10 Super-Secret Bonus Exercises No One Will Know you are Doing in Your Chair

For the past two years I have been creating customized office workouts for both businesses and individuals. Having worked with thousands of people, inevitably I run into the person who says "Oh, I'm not comfortable doing exercises in front of my coworkers," or "Public exercise? No way!" I try to be understanding and keep in mind that we each see life through different lenses. I'm going to try not to offend anyone here but I'm not going to make any promises because this kind of makes me crazy.

So what that person is saying is they aren't comfortable doing a few minutes of exercises in front of their fellow employees but they are comfortable with the prospect of developing a life-threatening disease, having to monitor their blood sugar throughout the day and inject insulin daily and live with the chance that they could go blind and/or lose a limb to gangrene. A few hip swivels at their desk would be outrageous but they are OK with the possibility of having to have major surgery followed by chemotherapy. A few biceps curls at the desk would be mortifying but they are perfectly content with walking around carrying 50 or 100 pounds of extra weight day in and day out. Having back pain is chill. Oh, and they are totally down with kicking the bucket 5 or 10 years before they have to. Honestly that kind of thinking mystifies me, but if that's you, I’ve created ten super-secret bonus exercises that can be done right in the comfort of your own chair that no one will ever know you are doing. These chair exercises are not nearly as effective as the 75 exercises that follow, but it beats doing nothing!

10 Super-Secret Bonus Exercises No One Will Know you are Doing in Your Chair

1. **Chest Squeeze:** Begin by sitting tall and upright in your seat with your core muscles engaged and spine elongated. Bring both hands in front of your chest with palms together and elbows pointing outward. Squeeze your palms together as hard as you can for 30 seconds. Rest and repeat at least once.
2. **Chest Pull:** Begin by sitting tall and upright in your seat with your core muscles engaged and spine elongated. Clasp hands firmly together in front of your chest keeping your palms pressed tightly together and elbows pointed outward. Then try to pull your hands apart as if someone were pulling on outward on each of your elbows, while keeping your hands firmly clasped. Sustain the pull for 30 seconds then repeat at least once.
3. **Hands Behind the Back Pull:** Begin by sitting tall and upright in your seat with your core muscles engaged and spine elongated. Bring your arms behind your back and clasp your right wrist with your left hand. Pull your shoulder blades together and downward as you try to pull your wrist out of your hand without actually releasing it. Hold the pull for 30 seconds and repeat at least once.
4. **Edge of Your Seat Abs:** Begin by sitting tall and upright in your seat with your core muscles engaged and spine elongated. Scoot your buttocks as far as you safely can towards the front edge of your chair. Place your hands on each side of the seat to help with stability (the less you hold on, the more challenging the exercise is). Lift you feet at least a few inches off the floor and hold that tall, seated position. Now round your spine towards the back of your chair (but don't touch your spine to the back of your chair). While keeping your feet off the floor, slowly return to the

tall seated posture. Repeat for 30 seconds, rest for a few seconds, and then do this exercise at least one more time.

5. **Butt Clench:** Begin by sitting tall and upright in your seat with your core muscles engaged and spine elongated. Yep, this is exactly what it sounds like: Just clench your buttocks firmly together and tighten the backs of your thighs. Hold the clench for 30 seconds, rest a few seconds, then repeat at least one more time.

6. **The Hover:** Begin by sitting tall and upright in your seat with your core muscles engaged and spine elongated. Place your hands firmly on the surface of your seat or on the surface of your armrests if they are strong and stable enough to hold your body weight. Push downward, lifting your body off of your seat and hover there for as long as you can. Repeat until you have hovered for at least a total of one minute.

7. **Leg Extensions:** Begin by sitting tall and upright in your seat with your core muscles engaged and spine elongated and feet firmly on the floor. Squeeze the insides of your thighs, knees and ankles tightly together. Then slowly extend your legs by lifting your feet off the floor and straightening the knees. When the legs are straight, squeeze the thighs tightly together, then slowly bend the knees and lower the feet to the floor. Repeat for one minute.

8. **Calf Raises:** Begin by sitting tall and upright in your seat with your core muscles engaged and spine elongated and feet firmly planted on the floor. Raise the heels up off the floor, coming up onto the balls of the feet. Squeeze the calves and the backs of your thighs tightly, then lower the heels back down. Repeat for one minute.

9. **Chair Rows:** (this exercise can only be done if you have a rolling chair): Begin by sitting tall and upright in your seat with your core muscles engaged and spine

elongated. Clasp the front edge of your desk with both hands (position hands slightly more than shoulder width apart), lift your feet off the floor and push slowly away as far as you can go, preferably until your arms are stretched and fully extended. Now pull yourself slowly back to the starting position and repeat for one minute.

10. **Crossover Pull:** Begin by sitting tall and upright in your seat with your core muscles engaged and spine elongated and feet firmly on the floor. Keep the feet and knees together. Place the left hand on the outside of the left thigh near the knee and with your right hand reach across your body and place your right hand on top of the left hand. Twist your torso to the right as if you were going to try to look over your right shoulder as you pull your hands firmly to the right. At the same time, press both thighs to the left, so they push firmly against the hands that are clasping them. Hold for 30 seconds and switch sides.

I recommend that you do at least one of these exercises per hour throughout your day. What we are trying to achieve here is 1-5 minutes of activity per hour.

8
25 Upper Body Strength Exercises using Resistance Bands

The exercises I'm about to describe are exercises that are easily done at your desk with a minimum of setup or interruption to your day. The size of a person's work space can vary from a closet to a corner office (don't laugh, I once had an office that was a cleaned out storage closet with a card table in it). You may not have enough room to do all of these exercises but I have tried to create a big enough variety of movements that you can get a workout no matter how much space you have.

There are a few safety precautions will need to take before doing these exercises. Take it from a guy who has been there and done that. You don't want a resistance band breaking and snapping in your face; always inspect the bands before you begin your exercises. Look for cuts or wear and tear in the bands and replace them if you see anything that looks like it could cause the band to break. Never… I repeat, NEVER use a band that looks like it might be damaged. Bands that are stored in your desk or office may have come in contact with sharp objects like scissors, letter openers, staplers etc and *must* be inspected before each use.

Always be aware of your surroundings. Make sure that you're not going to hit someone or something if you're swinging your arms or legs. If you have a band secured in a doorway, make sure that you have some way to let people know not to open the door. By following these simple safety procedures you can improve your health and not injure yourself or others in the process.

These 25 exercises are designed to improve muscle tone, increase strength, improve bone density, increase metabolism and help burn fat. As you get ready to do these exercises, you'll need to choose the correct resistance band for the type of muscle group you are working. Some muscles are bigger and more powerful than others.

Make sure that the band you are using for the exercise has enough resistance that the last 10 seconds of reps are very challenging. This will take a bit of experimentation with the individual exercises and your bands and workstation challenges. Don't get discouraged. And as you get stronger, you'll find that you'll be using the higher resistance bands more than the lower resistance bands. By the way, the description of each exercise comes first, followed by pictures of the exercise being performed. All of the cautions mentioned above apply to all 75 of the exercises in this book.

1. Lateral Raises

Grasp ends of resistance band. Stand with feet hip width apart and place center of band under each foot as an anchor. Holding handles of resistance bands in each hand, drop arms down to sides. Keeping arms bent, raise elbows and hands up until they reach shoulder height, and then lower them back to sides. Repeat for one minute.

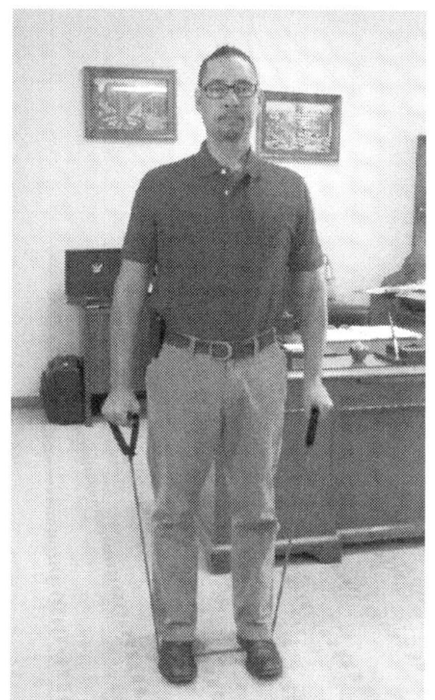

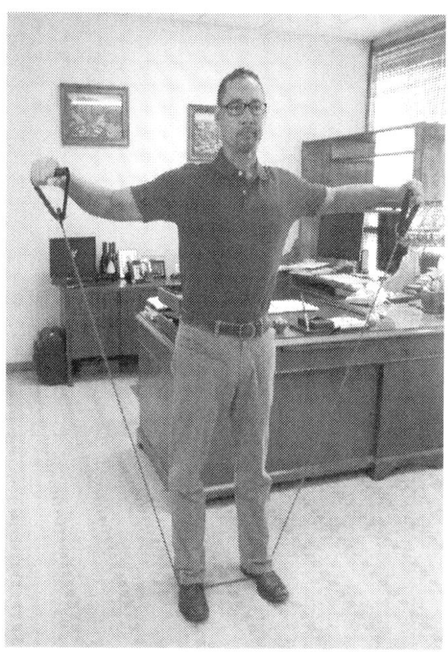

Lateral Raises

2. Front Raises

Grasp ends of resistance band. Stand with feet hip width apart and place center of band under each foot as an anchor. Holding handles of resistance bands in each hand, with hands down at your sides and palms facing backwards, lift both hands up with the palms facing down keeping the arms straight as you bring the hands to shoulder height. Lower the hands back down to your sides and repeat for one minute.

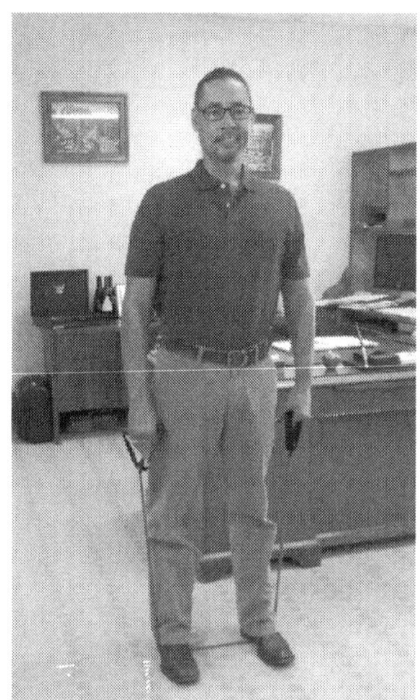

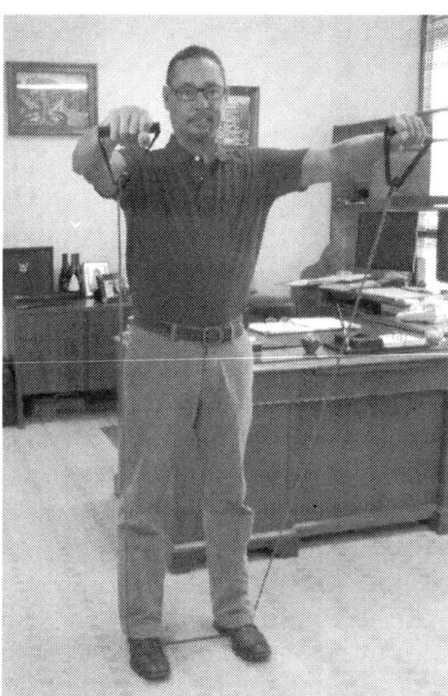

Front Raises

3. Shoulder Press

Grasp ends of resistance band. Stand with feet hip width apart and place center of band under each foot as an anchor. Holding handles of resistance bands in each hand, take arms out to sides and bend elbows. Hands should come to just above shoulders with palms facing upward as if supporting a tray in each hand while holding the handles of the resistance bands. Press hands up until arms are completely extended, then lower back down to complete the shoulder press. Repeat for one minute.

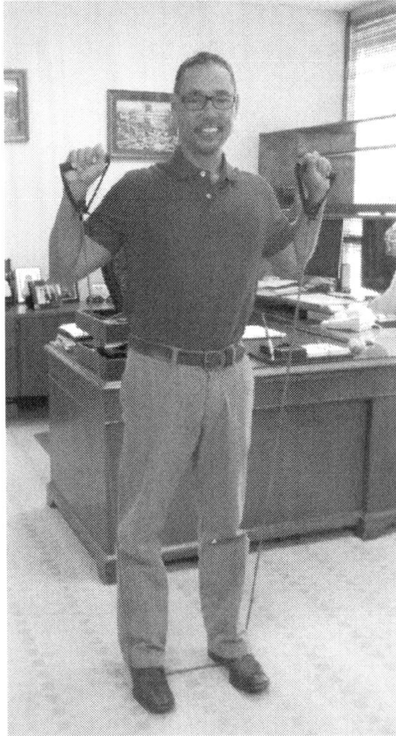

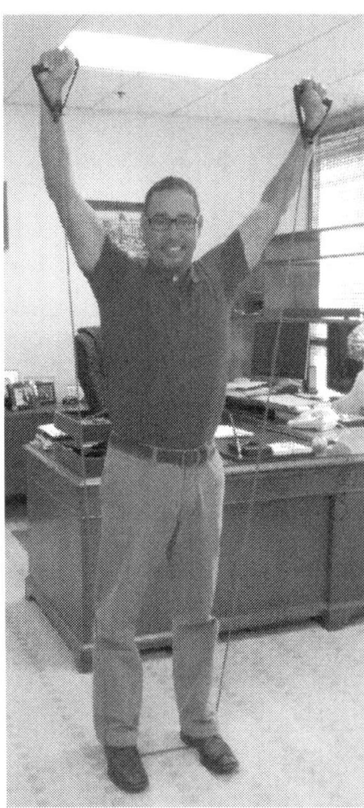

Shoulder Press

4. Wood Chop

Grasp handles of bands in each hand and step on the center portion of the bands. Still standing on the band, step feet out so that they are hip distance apart. Bring hands together and hold both handles at the same time with both hands. Bring both hands to the left side of the body. Pull the band across the body upwards towards the right shoulder. Return to original position. Repeat for 30 seconds, then switch sides and repeat for 30 seconds.

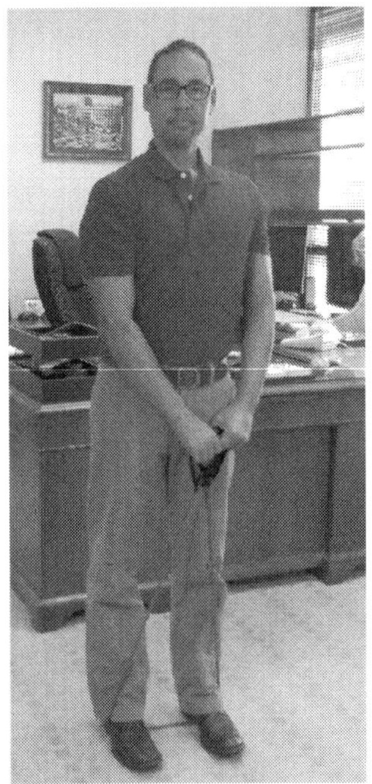

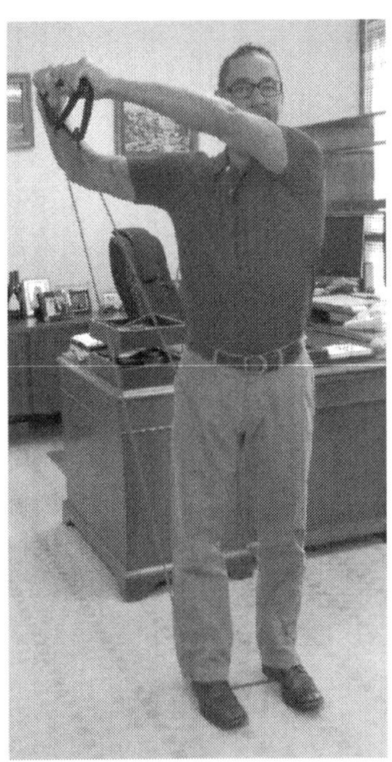

Wood Chop

5. Front Punch

Secure the bands in the door or to a stationary object at shoulder height. Turn your back on the door. Holding a handle in each hand, walk away until the band is tight and stand with the right foot in front of the left. Lean forward slightly. With both hands at shoulder height, palms down, fists facing forwards, punch forward with the right hand. Return to original position. Punch forward with left hand. Return to original position. Repeat, alternating hands, for one minute.

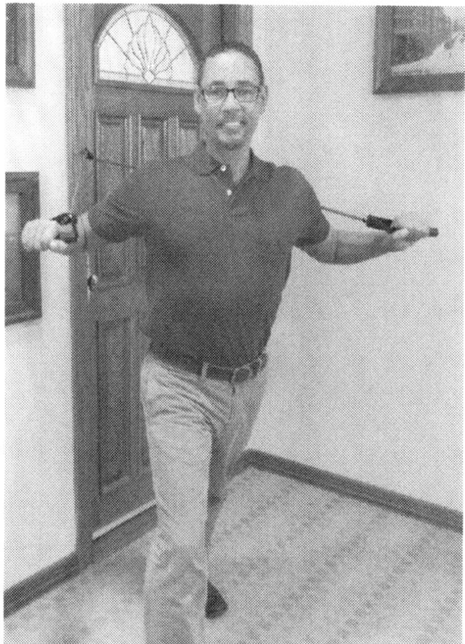

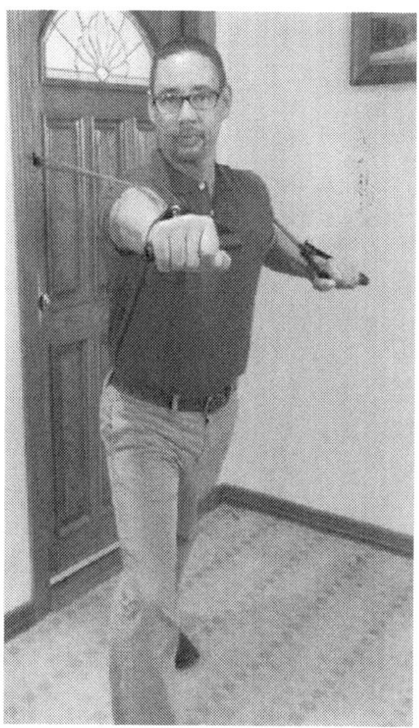

Front Punch

6. Biceps Curls

Grasp ends of resistance band and hold hands facing chest. Stand with feet hip width apart, and place center of band under each foot as an anchor. Keep wrists straight while holding hand bars palms are facing up. Don't bend wrists toward you or away from you. Maintain a slow, deliberate movement as you perform a bicep curl exercise with resistance band. Raise forearms toward you, and bend elbows to point where hands stop in front of shoulders. Hold handle at shoulder level for a second before releasing arms down. Release arms down, keeping palms facing up. Keep resistance band taut as you release hands to hip level. Maximum results will come from constant resistance of band during entire movement. Repeat for one minute.

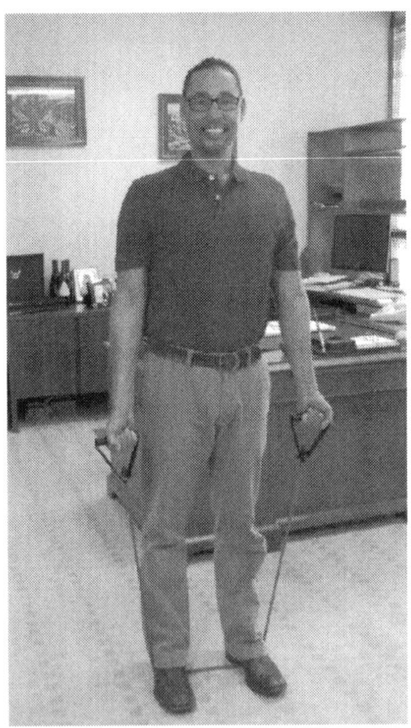

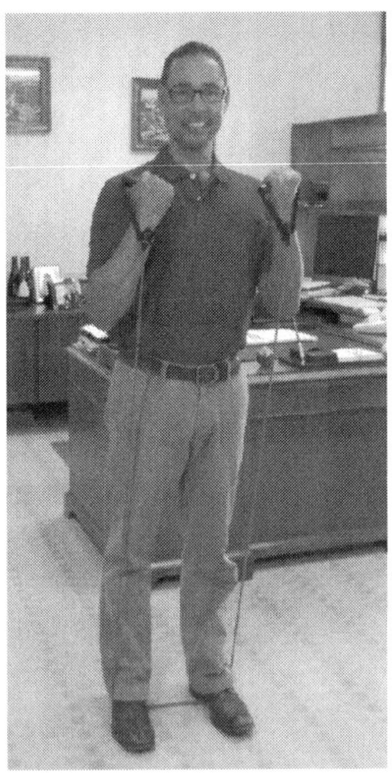

Biceps Curls

7. Concentration Curls (single hand)
While seated in a chair with both feet firmly planted on the ground, secure the center of the band around the right foot and hold both handles in the right hand, resting the right elbow on the right knee. Wrap roll the band around the right hand while still holding the handles until the band is tight when the hand is resting at knee level. Curl the right arm towards the right shoulder. Return to original position. Repeat for 30 seconds. Switch sides.

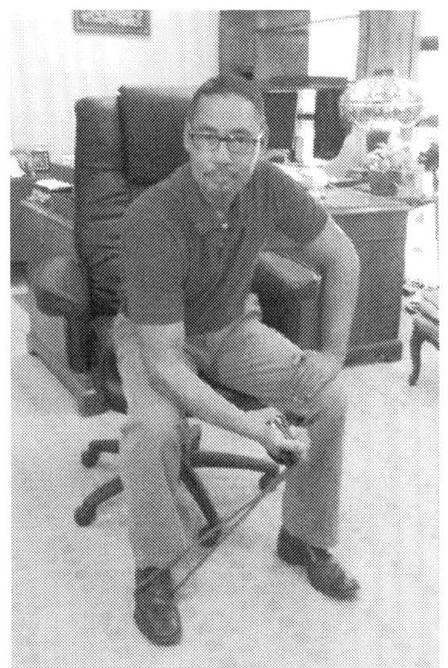
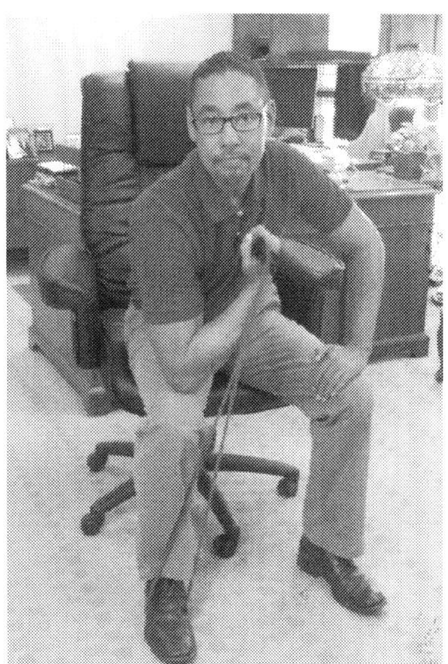

Concentration Curls (Single Hand)

8. Biceps Wing Curls

Grasp ends of resistance band. Stand with feet hip width apart and place center of band itself under both feet as an anchor. Keep wrists straight while holding hand bars. Don't bend wrists toward you or away from you. Rotate both arms outward then maintain a slow, deliberate movement as you pull both hands up towards shoulders. Hold hand bars at shoulder level for 1 second before releasing arms down. Release arms down, keeping hands facing outward. Keep resistance band taut as you release hands to hip level. Maximum results will come from constant resistance of band during entire movement. Repeat for one minute.

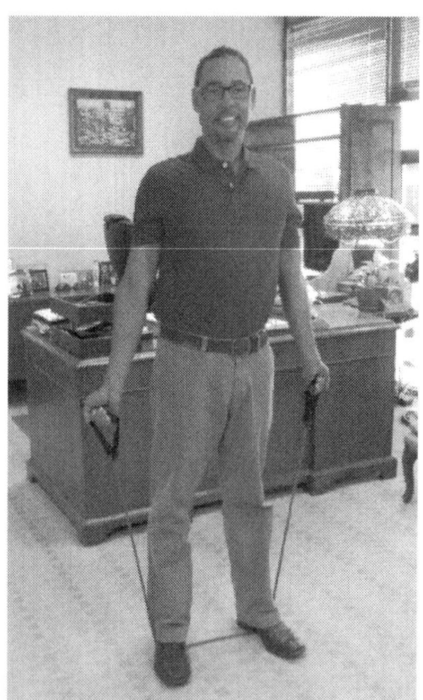

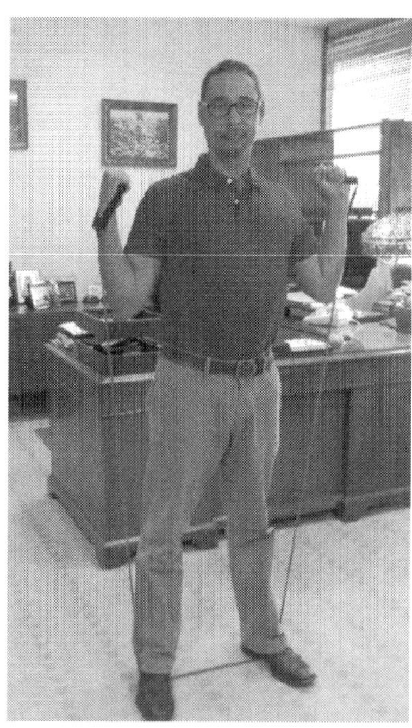

Biceps Wing Curls

9. Wing Curls (single hand)

Grasp ends of resistance band. Stand with feet hip width apart and place center of band itself under both feet as an anchor. Keep wrists straight while holding hand bars. Don't bend wrists toward you or away from you. Rotate both arms outward then maintain a slow, deliberate movement as you pull one hand up towards shoulders. Hold hand bar at shoulder level for 1 second before releasing arm down. Release arm down, keeping hand facing outward. Then repeat with other hand. Keep resistance band taut as you release hands to hip level. Maximum results will come from constant resistance of band during entire movement. Alternate between each hand for one minute.

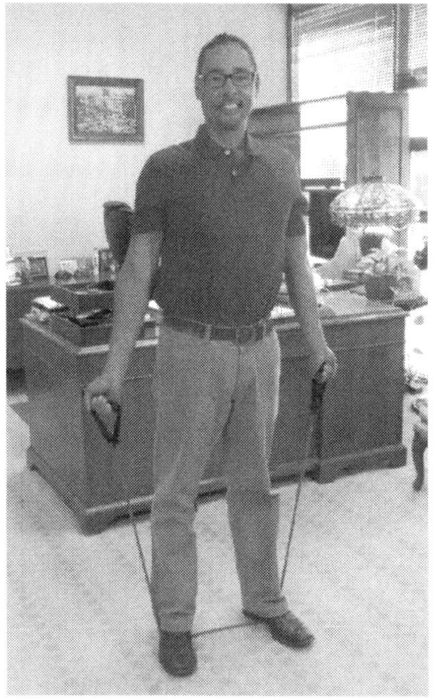

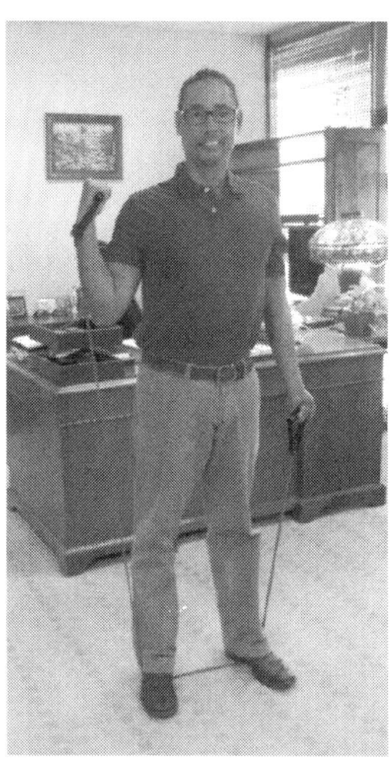

Wing Curls (single hand)

10. Hammer Curls

Grasp ends of resistance band and hold hands facing chest. Stand with feet hip width apart, and place center of band under each foot as an anchor. Bring the hands so that the palms face inward towards one another. Keep wrists straight while holding hand bars. Don't bend wrists toward you or away from you. Maintain a slow, deliberate movement as you perform a hammer curl exercise with resistance band. Raise forearms toward you, and bend elbows to point where hands stop in front of shoulders. Hold hand bars at shoulder level for a second before releasing arms down. Release arms down, keeping hands facing chest. Keep resistance band taut as you release hands to hip level. Maximum results will come from constant resistance of band during entire movement. Repeat for one minute.

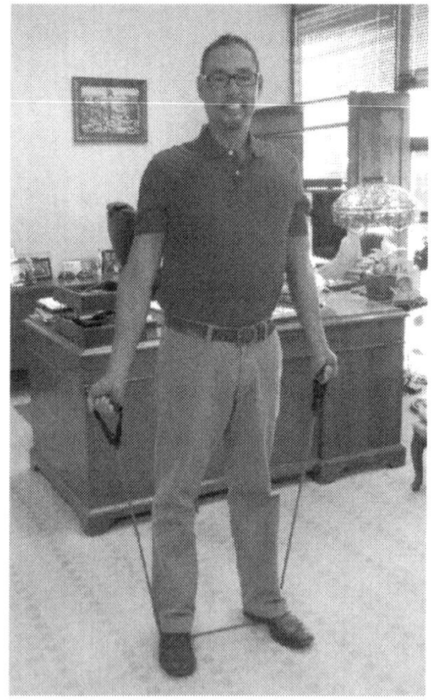

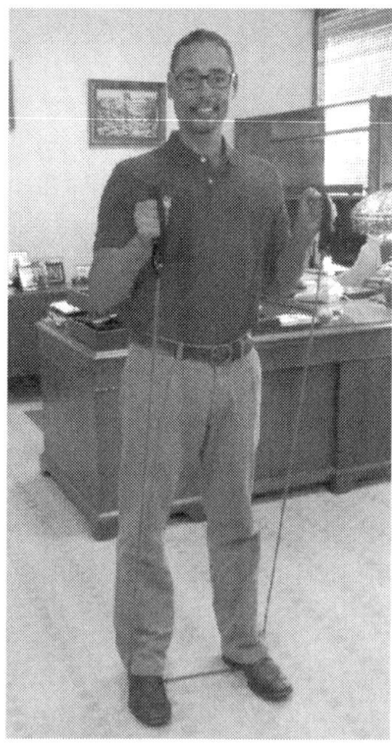

Hammer Curls

11. Reverse Curls

Grasp ends of resistance band and hold hands facing chest. Stand with feet hip width apart, and place center of band under each foot as an anchor. Bring the hands so that the palms face down towards the floor. Keep wrists straight while holding hand bars. Don't bend wrists toward you or away from you. Maintain a slow, deliberate movement as you perform a bicep curl exercise with resistance band. Raise forearms toward you, and bend elbows to point where hands stop in front of shoulders. Hold hand bars at shoulder level for a second before releasing arms down. Release arms down, keeping hands facing chest. Keep resistance band taut as you release hands to hip level. Maximum results will come from constant resistance of band during entire movement. Repeat for one minute.

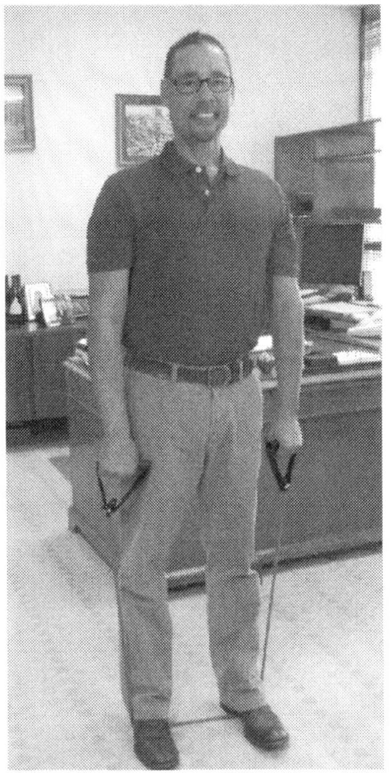

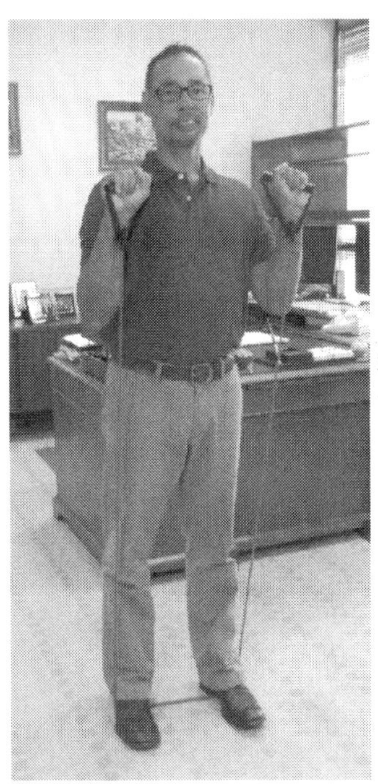

Reverse Curls

12. Chest Press

Anchor resistance band in a door or wrap it around a pole or other stationary object. Make sure resistance band will be lined up with middle of chest (i.e., band should run under arms). Stand in front of resistance band and grab both handles with an overhand grip. Walk away from object holding band until desired resistance is reached. Keep chest up, back straight and feet positioned with one foot in front of the other. Knees should have a slight bend. Having wrists aligned with elbows (straight forearm), press handles forward and bring them together at top of movement. Squeeze chest and hold for a count of 1. Lower handles back toward starting position in a slow and controlled manner, feeling stretch of pectoral muscles. Repeat for 50 seconds.

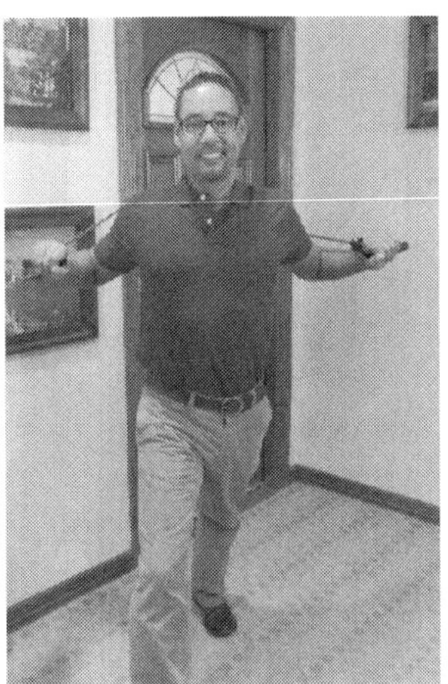

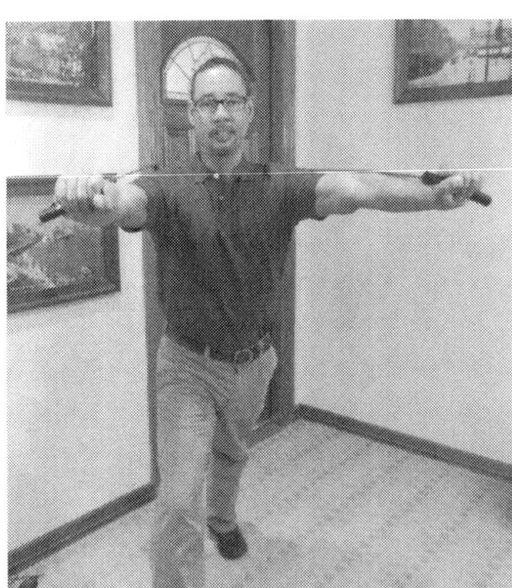

Chest Press

13. Chest Fly

Anchor band in a doorway or other stationary waist-high fixture and stand with back to band. Holding a handle in each hand, allow band to pull arms slightly behind you. Take a firm stance with one leg behind body for stability. Bring hands together in front of you, insides of fists almost touching. As you move, focus on chest muscles tensing as you bring hands together. Use a slow, controlled motion to get the most out of this exercise. Extend arms out to sides, roughly parallel with floor. Return to starting position, then repeat for one minute.

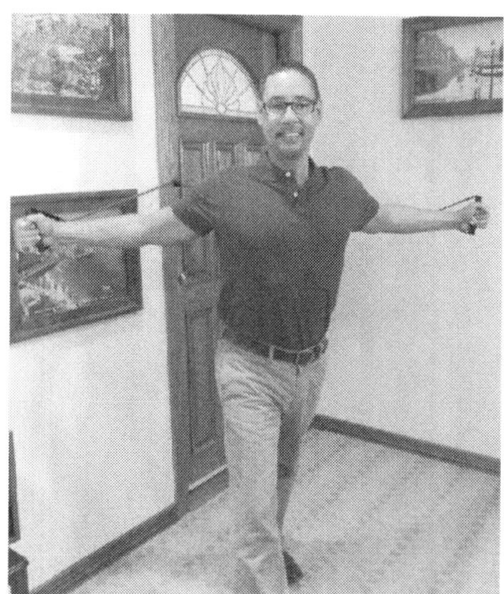
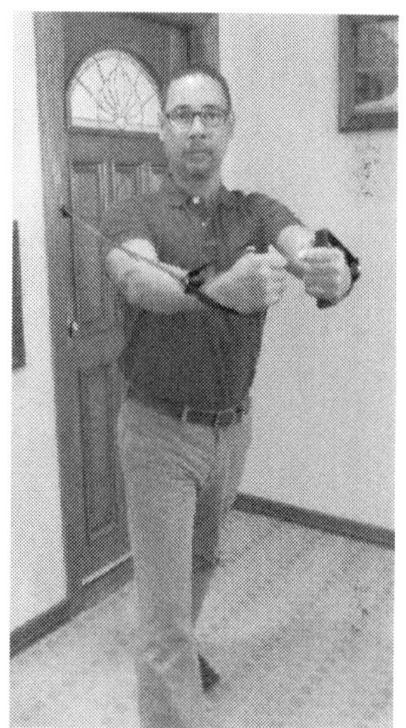

Chest Fly

14. Push Up

Grasp the band at each end so that the center of the band is behind your lower back and your hands are in front of you. Lie down in a push up position while still holding the band in each hand with your hands centered directly underneath your shoulders. The band should be tight at the lowest point of the push up and centered at your lower back, so as not to ride up to your neck at any point during the pushup. Press yourself up until your arms are fully extended, then slower lower back down to the original position, keeping the band tight. Continue for one minute, resting when needed.

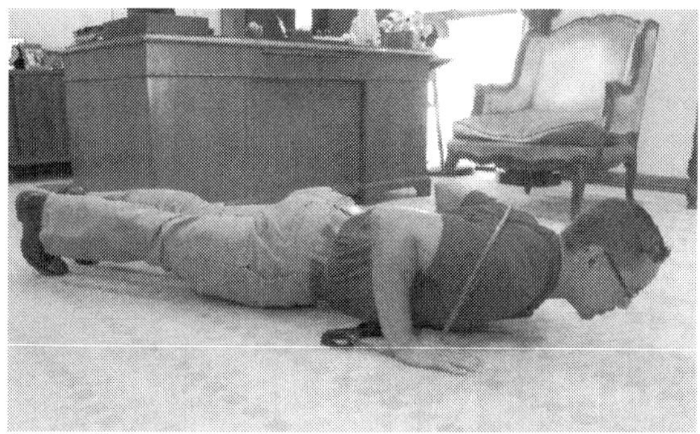

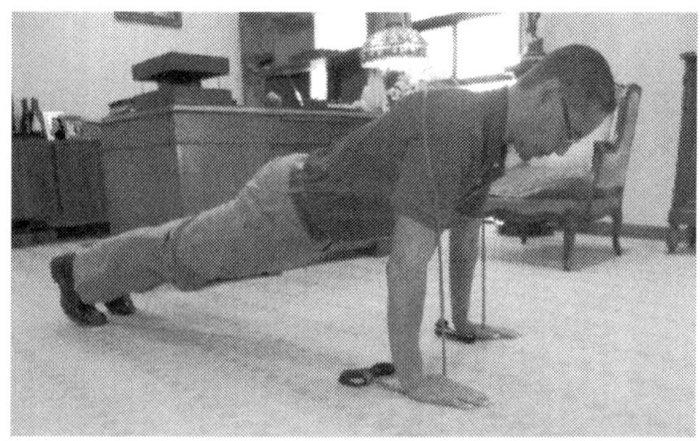

Push Up

Push Up, Continued

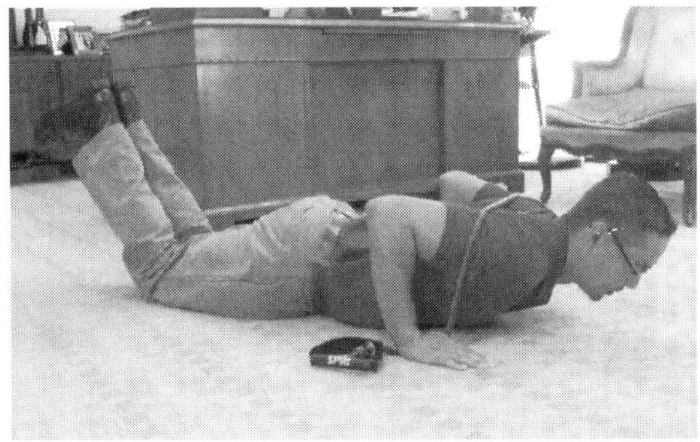

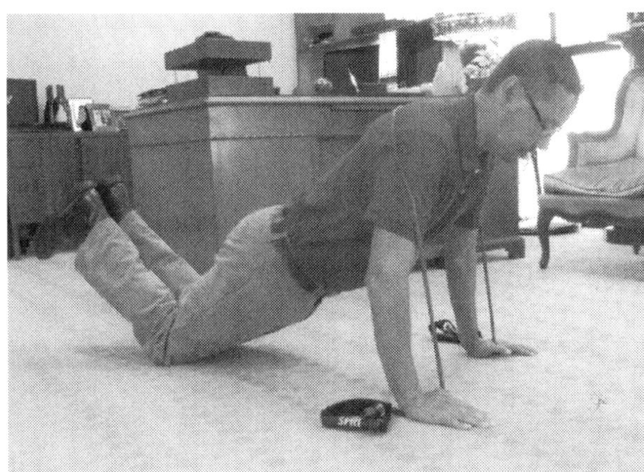

Push Up Modifications

15. The Hug

Secure the center of the band in the door or to a stationary object at waist height. Grasp the handles of the band in each hand and step away from the door until the band is free of slack. Place the right foot in front of the left and lean forward slightly. With arms extended and hanging at waist height, slightly away from the body, sweep both arms outwards and across the chest, in a motion similar to a bear hug. Finish with wrists crossed in front of the chest. Arms should stay extended throughout the motion. Return to original position. Repeat for one minute.

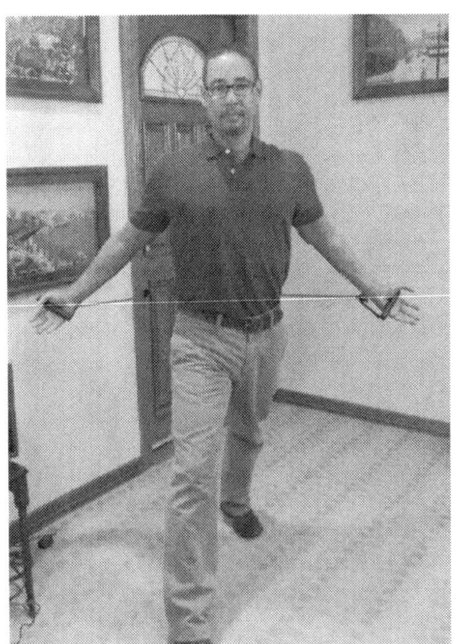

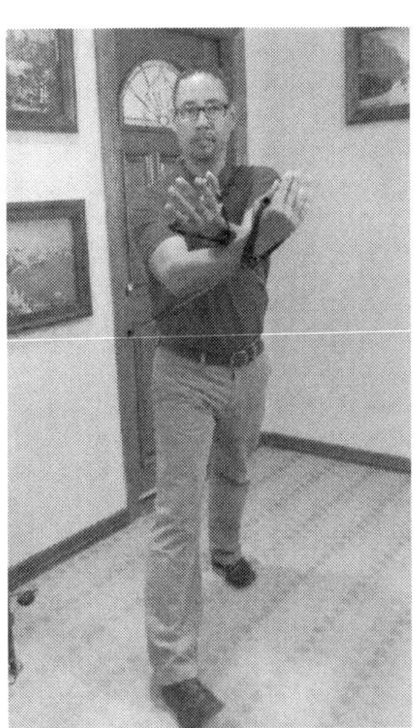

The Hug

16. Single Arm Chest Fly

Anchor band in a doorway or other stationary waist-high fixture and stand with back to band. Holding a handle in each hand, allow band to pull arms slightly behind you. Take a firm stance with one leg behind body for stability. Bring one arm in a sweeping motion, to the center line of the body with the palms facing towards the midline of the body. Return to original position, then repeat for 1 minute. Switch arms and repeat.

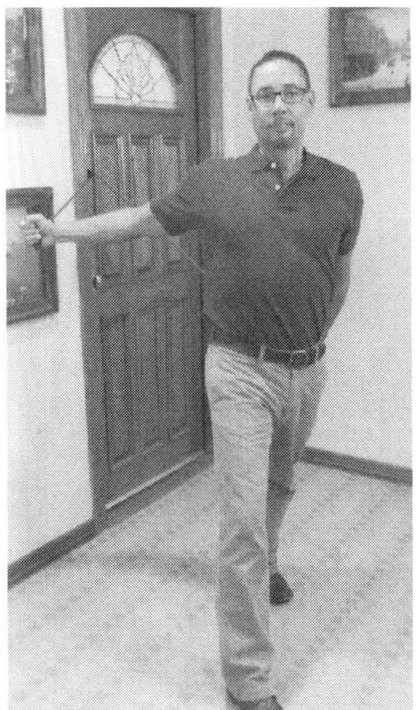

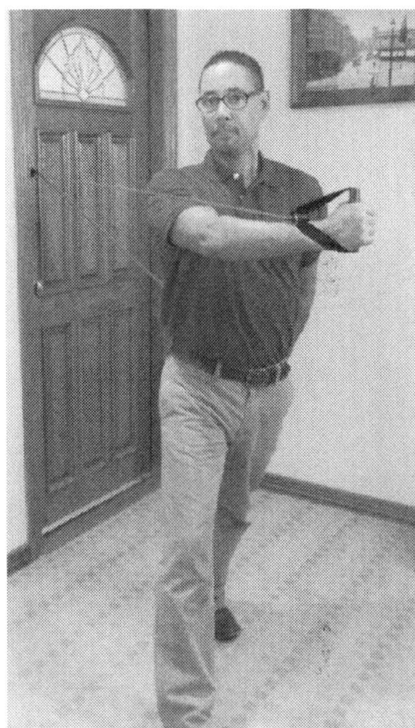

Single Arm Chest Fly

17. Wide Arm Push Up

Grasp the band at each end so that the center of the band is behind your lower back and your hands are in front of you. Lie down in a push up position while still holding the band in each hand with your hands well outside the shoulders. The band should be tight at the lowest point of the push up and centered at your lower back, so as not to ride up to your neck at any point during the pushup. Press yourself up until your arms are fully extended, then slower lower back down to the original position, keeping the band tight. Continue for one minute, resting when needed.

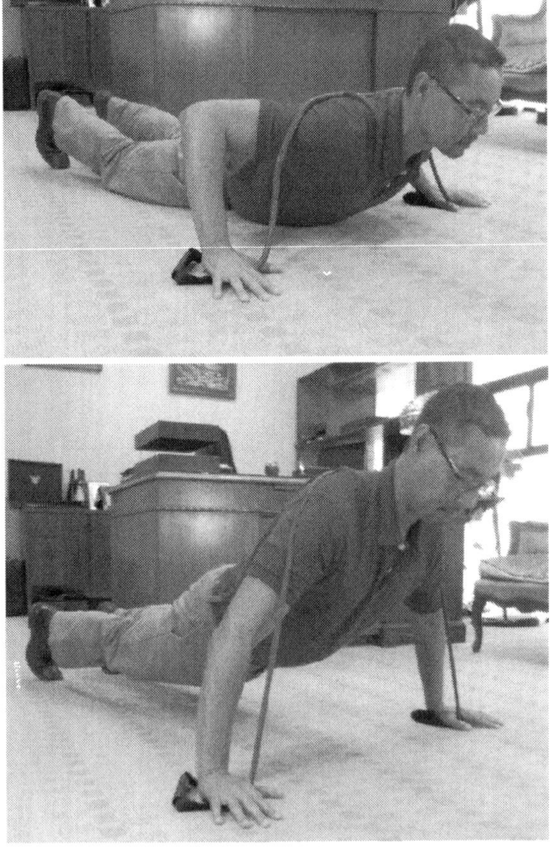

Wide Arm Push Up

18. Seated Row with Pulse

Secure the band in a door or to a stationary object at chest level while seated. Facing the anchor point, grasp a handle in each hand and sit far enough from the anchor point that the band is free of slack when your arms are fully extended in front of you. Engage your core, keeping your upper body still and upright. Bring arms back towards your chest, sweeping the elbows out and back until your hands are even with your upper chest. The motion should be similar to the action of rowing a boat with two oars. Now pulse backward three times, pulling the shoulder blades together at the same time. Repeat for 1 minute.

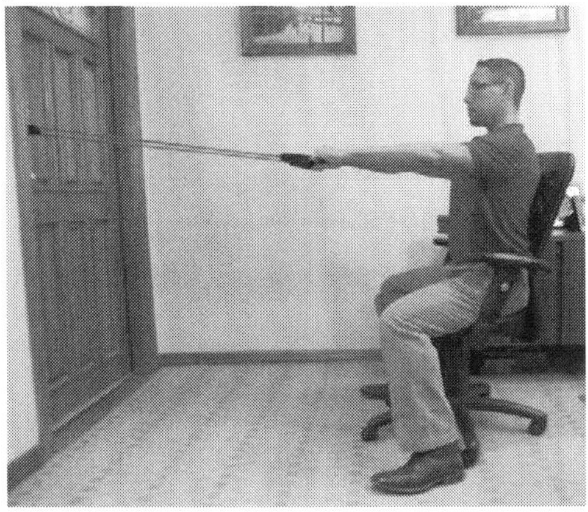

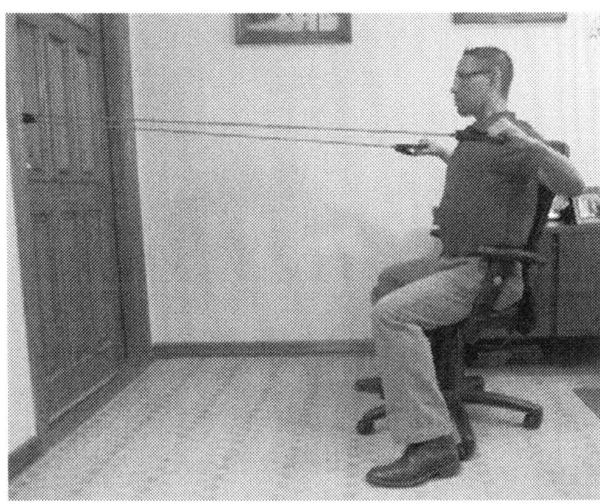

Seated Row with Pulse

19. Reverse fly

Secure the band in a door or to a stationary object at chest level while standing. Facing the anchor point, grasp a handle in each hand and step far enough away from the anchor point that the band is free of slack when your arms are fully extended in front of you. Place your right foot in front of your left and, keeping your arms and back straight, engage your core and bring your arms out to your sides at shoulder height. This motion is similar to the hug, only in reverse and without crossing the wrists.

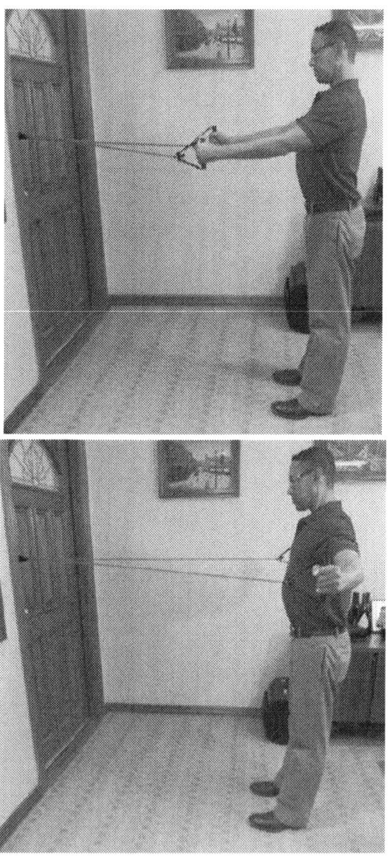

Reverse Fly

20. Lat Pull-down

Secure the center of the band in the top of a doorway or to a stationary object at a comparable height. Facing the anchor point, step back until the band is free of slack and grasp a handle in each hand at shoulder height or slightly higher. Pull back towards your body and downward bending the elbows slightly so that the ending position of your hands leaves them even with the body between the lower ribs and hips. Return to original position. Repeat for one minute.

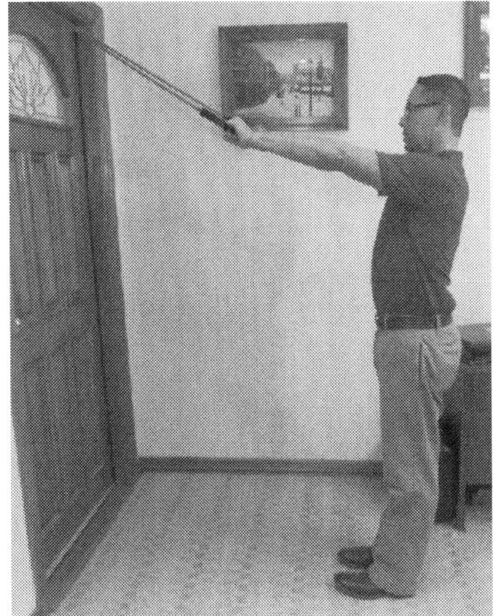
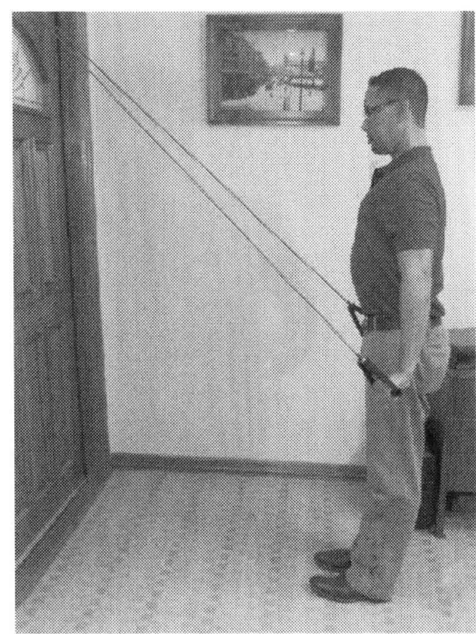

Lat Pull-down

21. Shrug

Holding one handle in each hand, stand on the center of the band with both feet. Both feet should be together and back should be straight. Grasp the band in each hand in a location that leaves the band free of slack when your arms are extended at your sides. Depending on your height and the length of the band you may need to grasp it below the handles. With your feet together, arms extended and back straight, shrug your shoulders, bringing them up towards your ears. Return to starting position. Repeat for one minute.

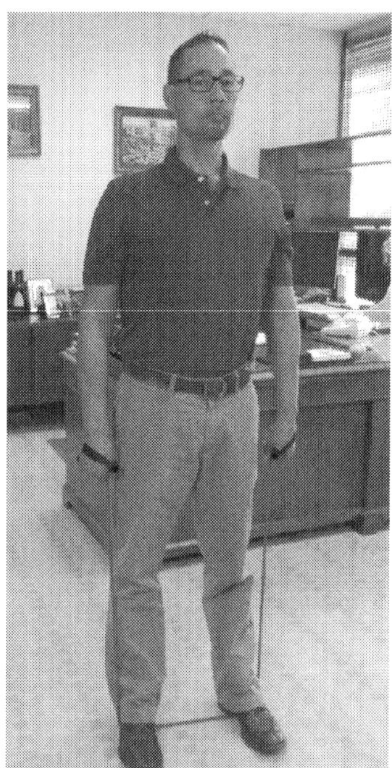
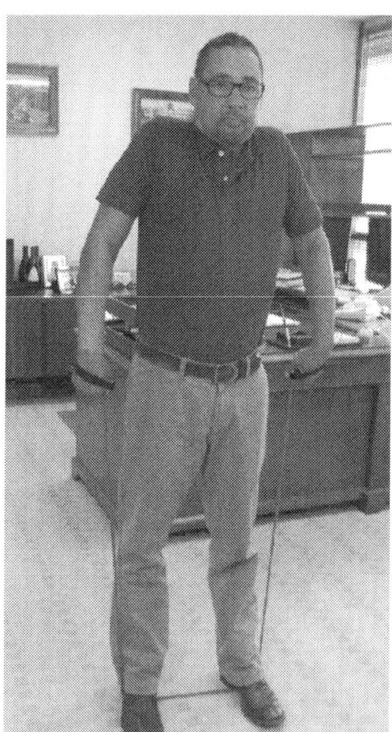

Shrug

22. Bent Over Row (Two-Handed)

Stand on the center of the band with your feet hip distance apart. Holding one handle in each hand, bend your knees slightly and lean forward at the waist, until your upper torso is parallel to the ground. Look directly down at the floor keeping the neck in line with the rest of the back. Your elbow should be bent and angled to the sides and the band should be taught when the fists are in line with the knees. Bring arms back towards your chest, sweeping the elbows out and back until your hands are even with your upper chest. The motion should be similar to the action of rowing a boat with two oars. Repeat for 1 minute.

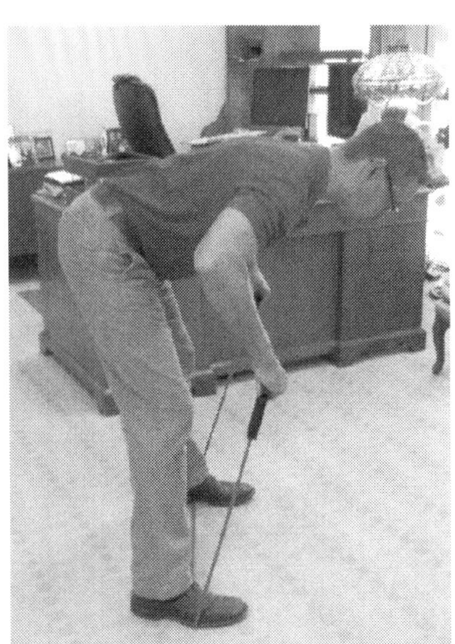

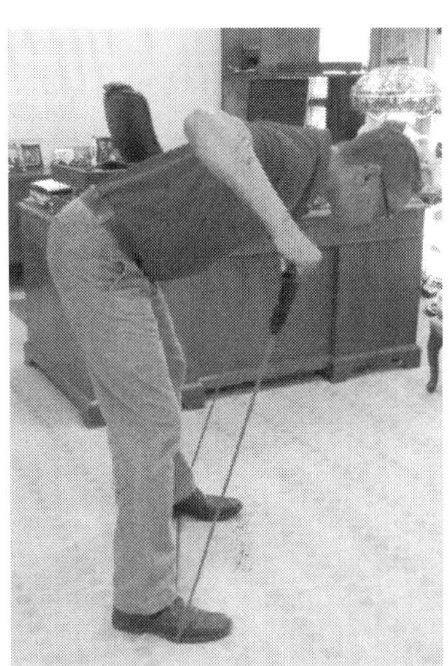

Bent Over Rows (Two-Handed)

23. Bent Over Row (Single Handed)

Stand on the center of the band with your feet hip distance apart. Holding one handle in each hand, bend your knees slightly and lean forward at the waist, until your upper torso is parallel to the ground. Look directly down at the floor keeping the neck in line with the rest of the back. Your elbow should be bent and angled to the sides and the band should be taught when the fists are in line with the knees. Bring one arm back towards your chest at a time, sweeping the elbow out and back until your hand are even with your upper chest. Alternate hands. The motion should be similar to the action of rowing a boat with two oars. Repeat for 1 minute.

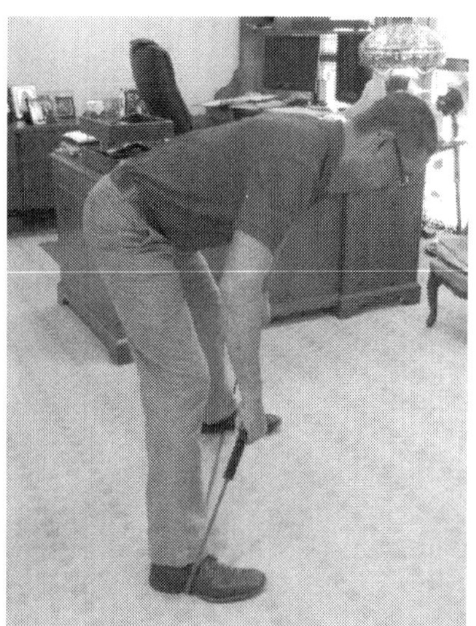

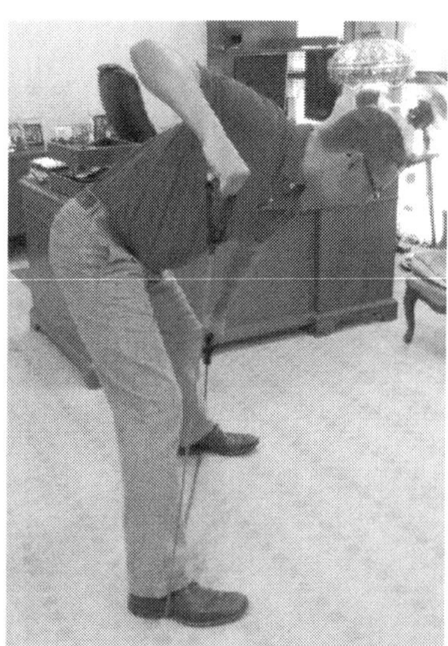

Bent Over Row (Single Handed)

24. Reverse Starfish

Secure the center of the band in the top of the doorway or to a stationary object of a comparable height. Face the anchor point and grasp one handle in each hand. Step back so that the band is free of slack when both arms are extended at shoulder level. Your feet should be parallel to the doorway, shoulder width apart. Engaging your core, keeping both arms extended pull down in a sweeping motion towards your hips with both hands simultaneously. Continue until your hands are past your hips, behind you. Return to starting position. Repeat for one minute.

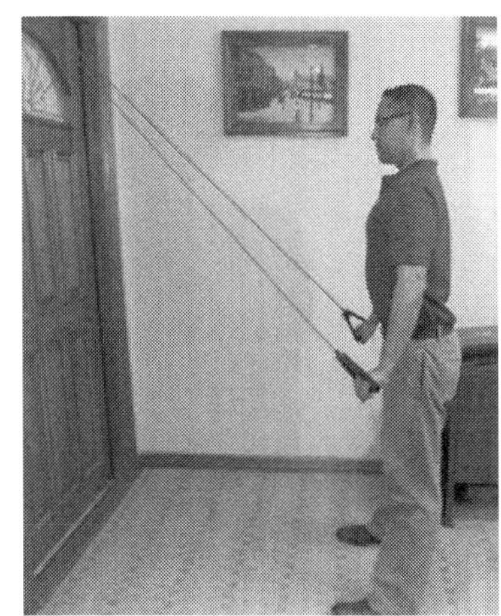
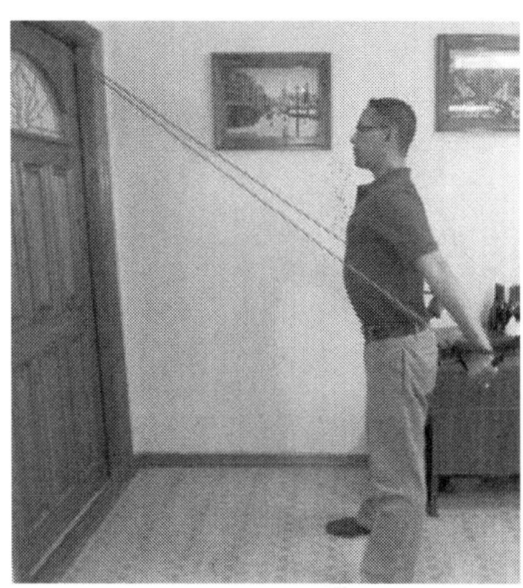

Reverse Starfish

25. Scaption

Grasping one handle in each hand, stand on the center of the band with one foot and step back one step with the other. Keep your hips squared and your chest facing the same direction as your forward foot. With your arms extended, raise them out in front of you at an angle until they are at shoulder height and slightly further than shoulder width apart. At the full extension, your fists should be pointed forwards like you are holding onto ski poles, and the band should be forming a 30 degree V shape. Return to starting position. Repeat for one minute.

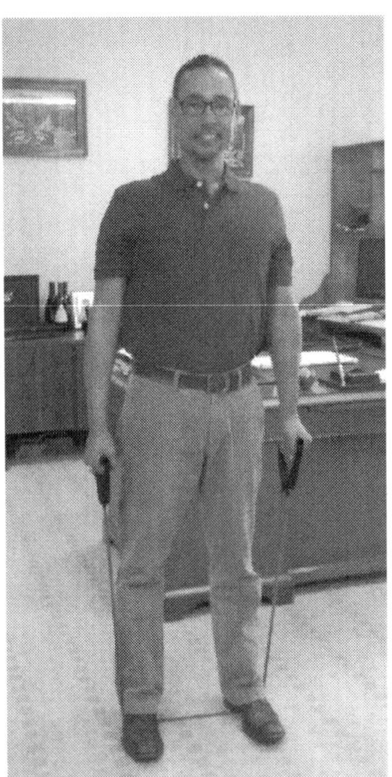
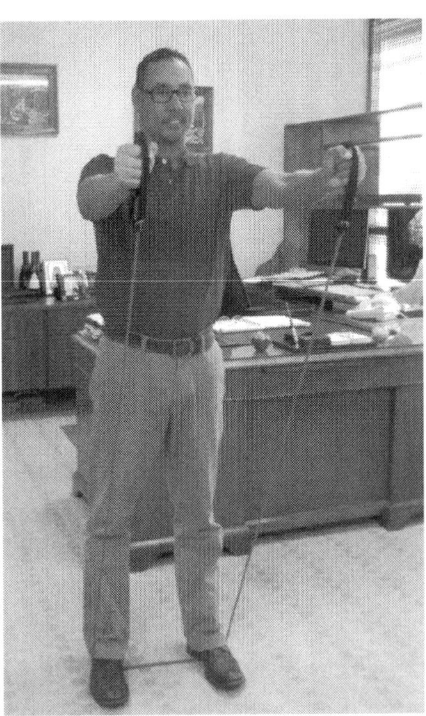

Scaption

9
The Upper Body Strength Program

3-Day Upper Body Strength Program

I have created a sample three day upper body strength training program for the office. This program was designed for people who only want to work on upper body strength. For those of you who are new to strength training, you may wonder why I am only recommending 3 days of upper body strength training per week. I do this because it is important to allow the muscles to rest between strength training sessions. This allows the muscles to grow and allows the body to recover. In a perfect world, you would give yourself one full day of "rest" between training sessions. Having said that, few of us live in perfect worlds, and working out back to back days shouldn't do any serious harm. But remember that rest is equally as important as the workout.

In order to be sure you stay on schedule, just set an alarm on your smart phone or on your daily Outlook calendar to remind you it's time for your 5 minute workout. You'll notice in the "schedules" below that I have you doing your workout at 45 minutes past the hour; that was entirely arbitrary. Create the schedule that works best for you and your workplace. Just keep in mind that you really need to get up and get moving each and every hour.

Each of the exercises listed below should be done for exactly one minute. If you decide to do all five exercises each hour, you should be back to work after no more than five minutes. (If you are pressed for time in any given hour, just do 2 or 3 of the exercises and get back to work!)

Day 1

9:45

- Lateral raises
- Biceps curls
- Standing chest press
- Seated row with Pulse
- Shrug

10:45

- Scaption
- Concentration Curls
- Push Up
- Reverse Fly
- Wood Chop

11:45

- Front Raises
- Wing Curls
- Chest Flys
- Lat Pulldown
- Reverse Starfish

1:45

- Shoulder presses
- Reverse Curls
- Single Arm Chest Fly
- Bent Over Row
- The Hug

2:45

- Front Punch
- Hammer Curls
- Wide Arm Push Up
- Bent Over Row (single handed)
- Wing Curl (single handed)

Day 2

10:45

- Front Raises
- Concentration Curls
- Wide Arm Push Up
- Shrug
- Wood Chop

11:45

- Front Punches
- Wing Curls
- The Hug
- Reverse Fly
- Reverse Star fish

1:45

- Lateral Raises
- Reverse Curls
- Chest Fly
- Seated Row with Pulse
- Scaption

2:45

- Front Raises
- Concentration Curls
- Single Arm Chest Fly
- Lat Pull Down
- Bent Over Row (single handed)

3:45

- Wood Chop
- Front Punch
- Hammer Curls
- Push Up
- Bent Over Row

Day 3

9:45

- Reverse Starfish
- Wide Arm Push Up
- Reverse Curls
- Scaption
- Wood Cop

10:45

- Lateral Raises
- Biceps Curls
- Standing Chest Press
- Seated Row with Pulse
- Shrug

11:45

- Bent Over Row (single handed)
- Single Arm Chest Fly
- Hammer Curls
- Scaption
- Front Punches

1:45

- Front Raises
- Concentration Curls
- The Hug
- Bent Over Row (two handed)
- Lat Pull Down

2:45

- Shoulder Presses
- Wing Curls
- Chest Fly
- Seated Row with Pulse
- Reverse Starfish

10
25 Lower Body Strength Exercises

The exercises I'm about to describe are exercises that are easily done at your desk with a minimum of setup or interruption to your day.

These exercises are for the muscles of the lower body. These muscles are very important because they are the foundation upon which your body is built. Nearly 65% of your muscles are in your lower body. The muscles in your lower body are also some of the largest muscles in the body. This makes building the muscles of the lower body important for weight loss since these big muscles increase metabolism.

Make sure that the band you are using for the exercise has enough resistance that the last 10 seconds of reps are very challenging. This will take a bit of experimentation with the individual exercises and your bands and workstation challenges. Don't get discouraged. And as you get stronger, you'll find that you'll be using the higher resistance bands more than the lower resistance bands.

1. Chair Squats:
Begin by sitting on a chair with feet hip distance apart. Your knees should be aligned directly over your ankles. Sit up tall and bring your arms out in front of you at shoulder height with the palms of your hands pointed in towards the center line of your body. Stand, then drop the buttocks down as if to sit, trying to keep as much weight *off* the chair as you can when coming down to the seated position. Press back up to the original position. Repeat for one minute.

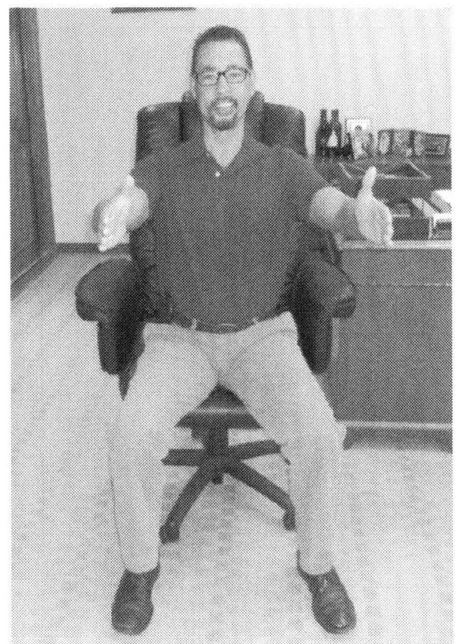

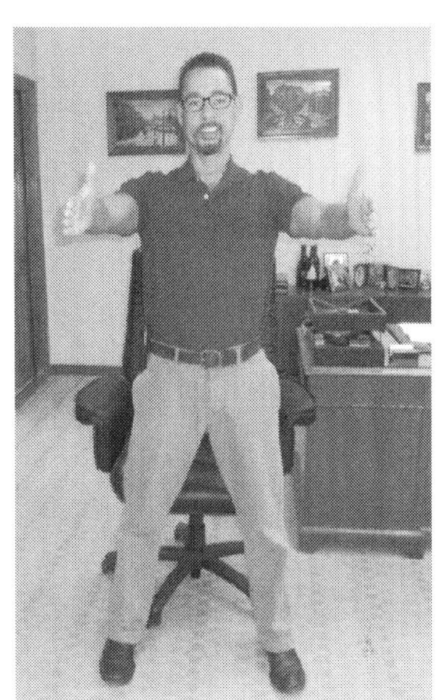

Chair Squats

2. Single Leg Rolling Lunges: Begin standing facing your desk. Grab a hold of the desk for balance Place one leg up on your exercise ball so that soul of the foot is pressed lightly against the front of the ball holding it in place. Align front foot forward so you are in a lunging position. Keeping hips rolled under, bend the front knee down as you roll the ball back and away from you slowly lowering your hips down towards the ground.When the ball has been pushed as far back as you can and still keep it under your foot pause then pull the ball back to the starting position as you press back up. Do on one side for 25 seconds, then switch to opposite side for 30 seconds**.**

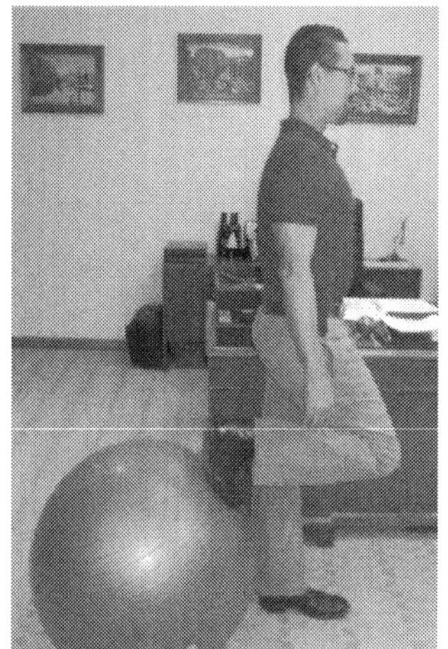

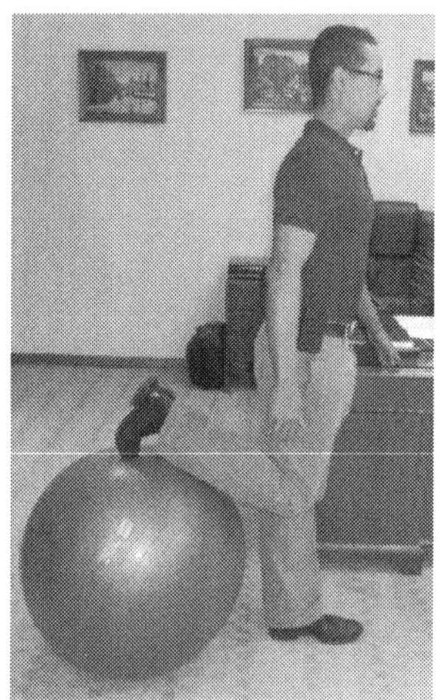

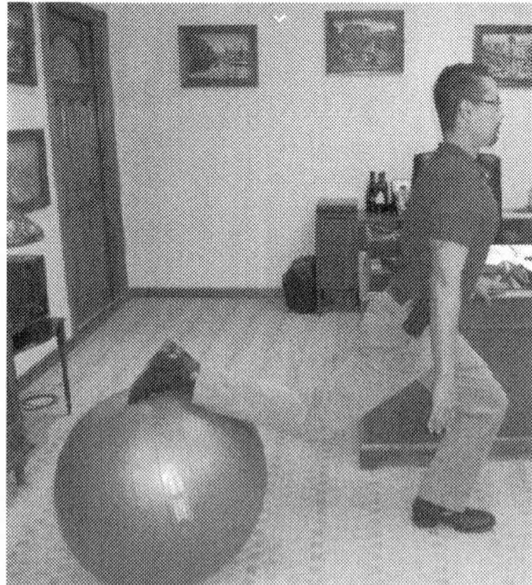

Single Leg Rolling Lunges

3. Wall Squats: Stand facing away from a clear wall surface with your back against the wall and feet about 12-18" away from the wall. Press back firmly into wall. Slide down until knees are at about 90-degree angles (or an angle that is comfortable for you) and hold, keeping abs contracted, for one minute.

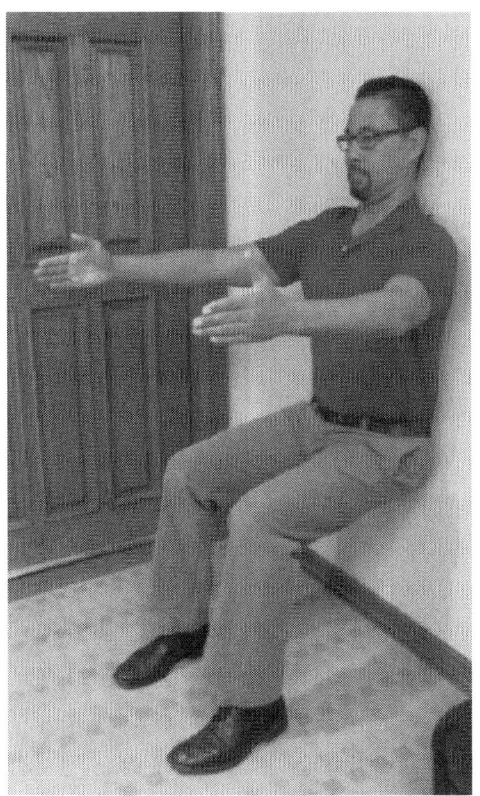

Wall Squats

4. The Kick: Attach both ends of the band to a stationary object near the ground. Loop the band around your ankle and face away from the object the band is attached to keeping the band taught. Slowly kick the leg forward then return to the original position repeat for 30 seconds then switch legs.

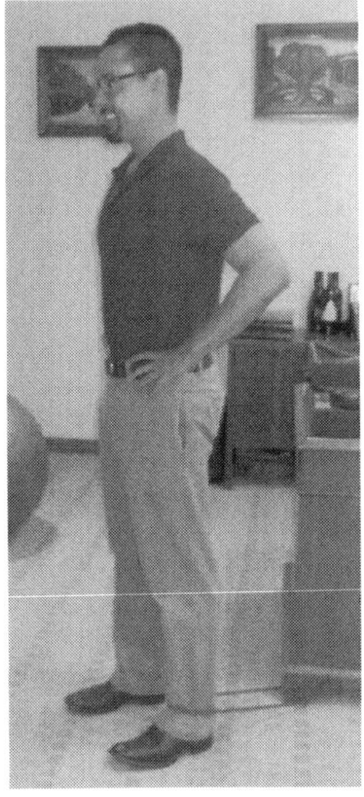

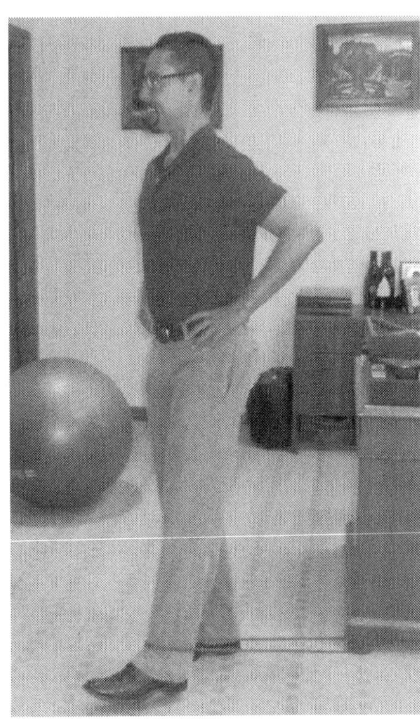

The Kick

5. Tush Tightener: Attach both ends of the band to a stationary object near the ground. Loop the band around your ankle and face the object the band is attached to keeping the band taught. Slowly kick the leg backwards then return to the original position repeat for 30 seconds then switch legs.

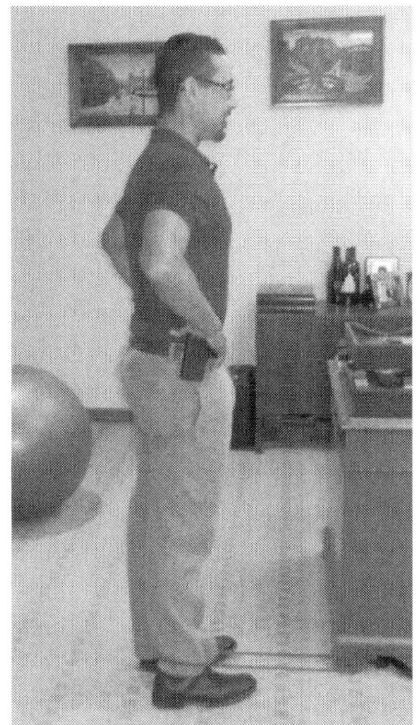
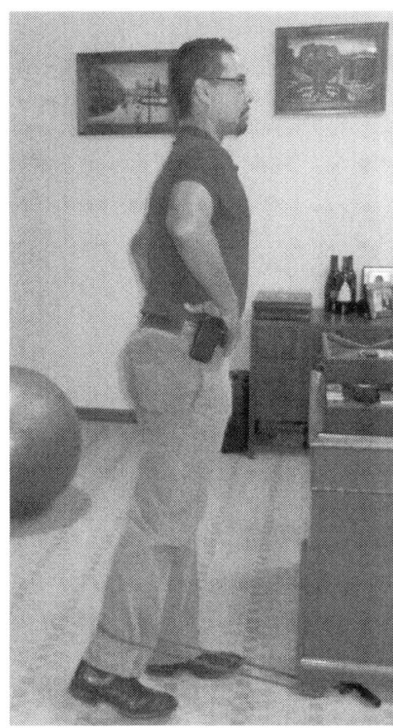

Tush Tightener

6. Side Beats: Attach both ends of the band to a stationary object near the ground. Loop the band around your right ankle keeping the band taught. With the stationary object securing the band at your left, stand with your feet hip distance apart. Place your left hand on your desk or chair to steady yourself then shift all your weight onto your left foot, keeping your torso erect and spine tall. Swing your right leg sideways (out to the right of your body) as you point the toe. Lift your foot anywhere from 1 to 12 inches off the floor (the higher you lift the leg the more difficult the movement). Drop your foot down to the floor and lightly touch the toe on the ground then lift it again. Repeat for 30 seconds then switch sides.

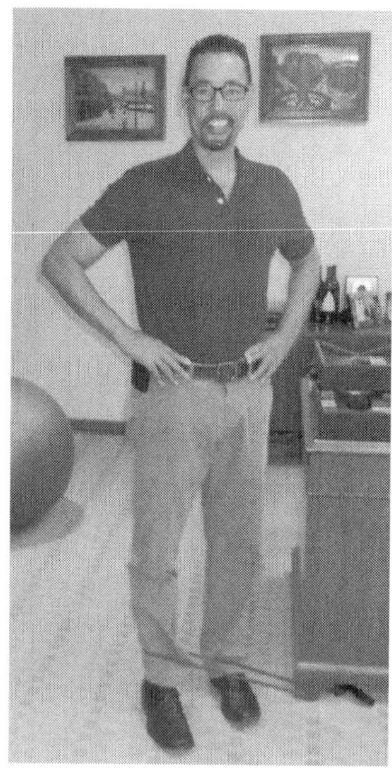
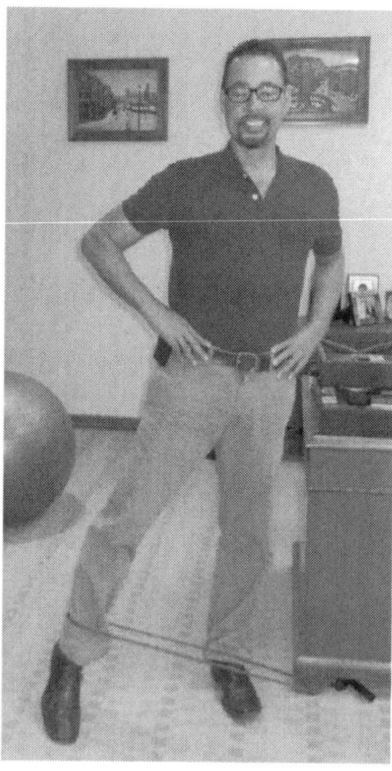

Side Beats

7. Crossovers: Attach both ends of the band to a stationary object near the ground. Loop the band around your right ankle keeping the band taught. Stand with your feet hip distance apart with your left desk or a chair that will not move directly to your right. Place your right hand on your desk or chair to steady yourself then shift all your weight onto your left foot, keeping your torso erect and spine tall. Swing your right leg across your body and out to the left as you point the toe. Return to your original position. Repeat for 30 seconds then switch sides.

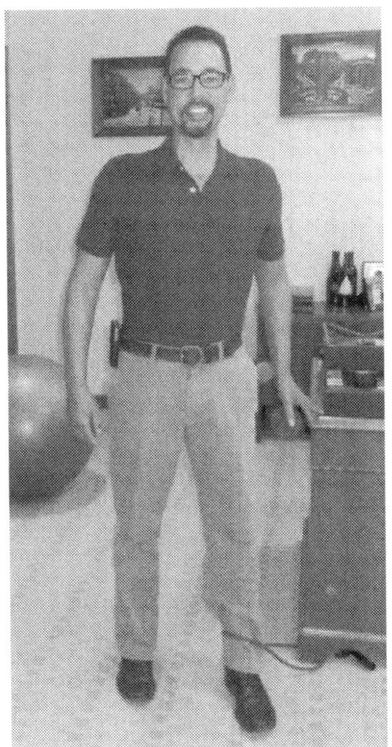

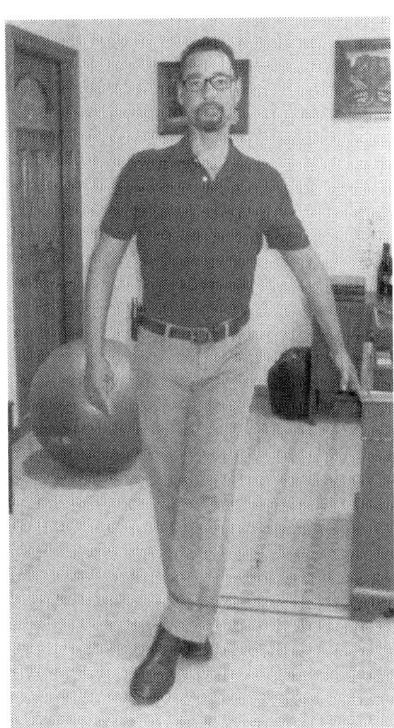

Crossovers

8. Seated Ball Hamstring Curls (single leg): Sitting in a chair, place one foot on an exercise ball (your leg should be fully extended). Press your heel firmly down into the ball then pull the ball towards you trying to keep the ball moving in a straight line and pushing down hard into the ball with your heel. Press the leg away returning the ball to its original position. Repeat for 30 seconds then switch legs.

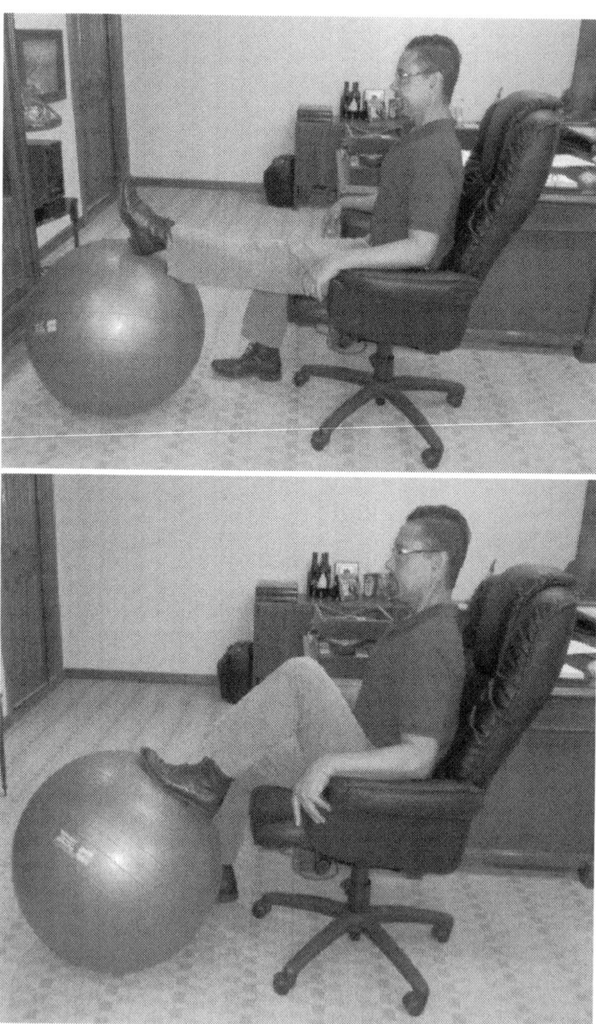

Seated Ball Hamstring Curls (single leg)

9. Touch Down: Stand next to your desk or other stationary object. Place one hand on the desk or object to aid in balance then lift one foot off the ground as you balance on the other foot. Slowly bend the knee of the leg you are standing on as you reach down to touch the floor, dropping the buttocks down towards the ground and bending forward at the waist as little as possible. After touching the ground return to starting position without pushing with the hand that is on the desk to help you up. Repeat for 30 seconds then switch legs.

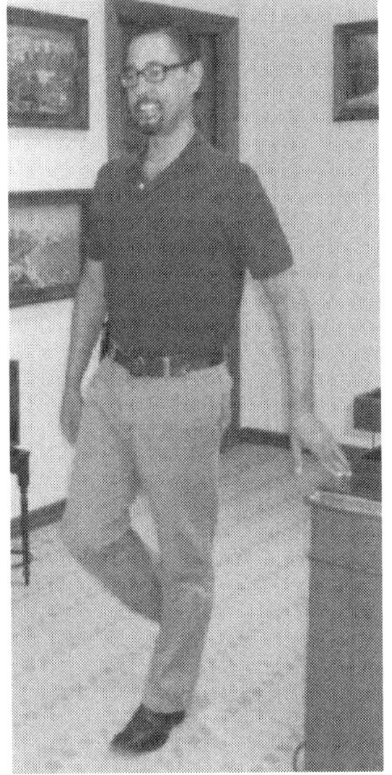

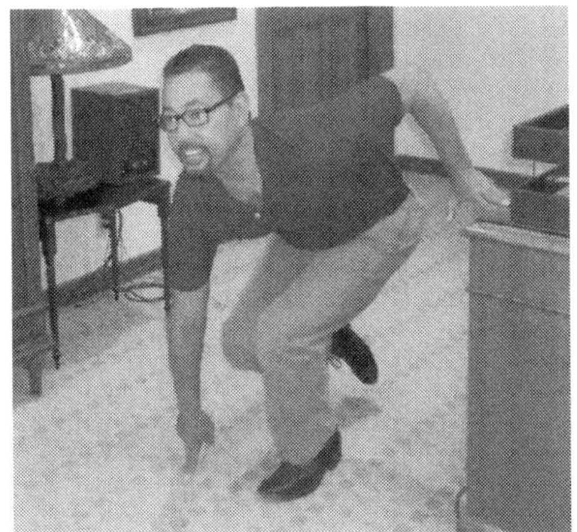

Touch Down

10. Curtsy Squat: Stand with your feet hip distance apart. Step back and to the left with your right foot as far as you can safely, crossing your right leg behind your left leg as you bend both knees lowering your body down towards the ground. Return to original position and repeat for 30 seconds then switch sides.

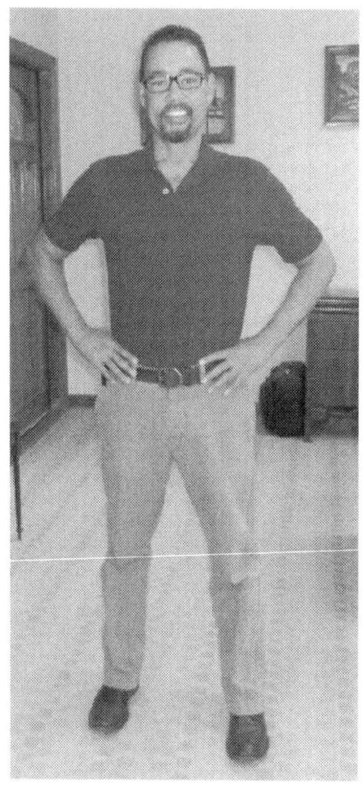

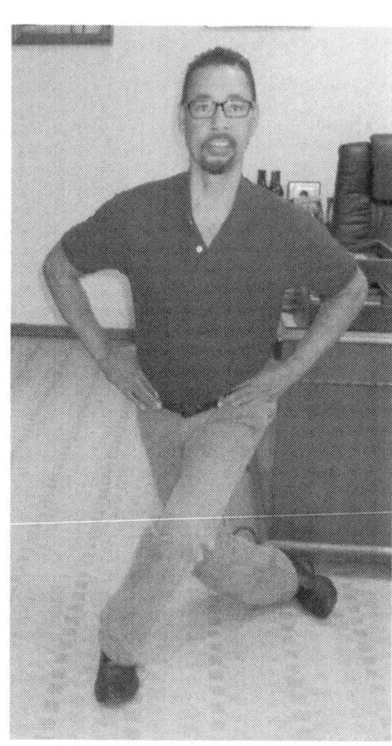

Curtsy Squat

11. Wide Leg Squat: Stand with your arms folded at your chest. Spread your legs so they are twice hip distance apart with toes pointed forward. Bend your knees as you drop your buttocks down towards the floor as if you were going to sit in a chair, but be sure to keep your torso as upright as possible. Then return to the starting position. Repeat for one minute.

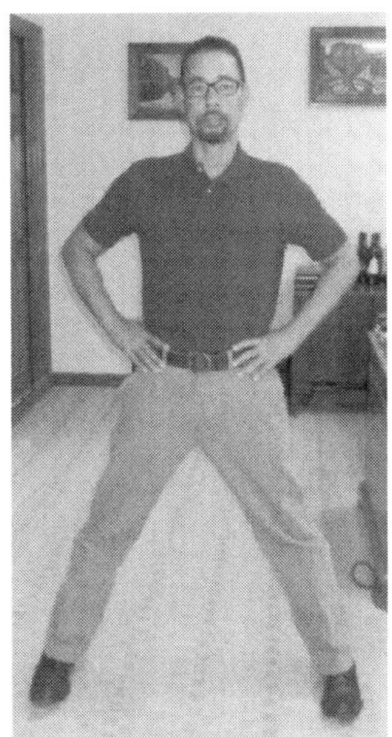

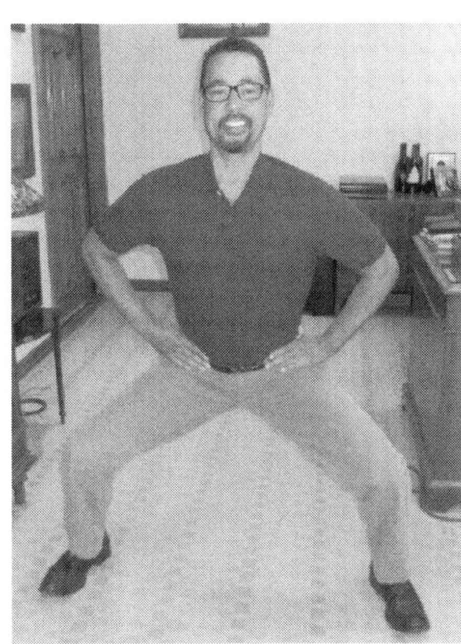

Wide Leg Squat

12. Calf Raises: Stand with your feet hip distance apart. Rise up onto your toes as high as you can then gently contract your calf muscle. Lower back down to your starting position. Repeat for one minute.

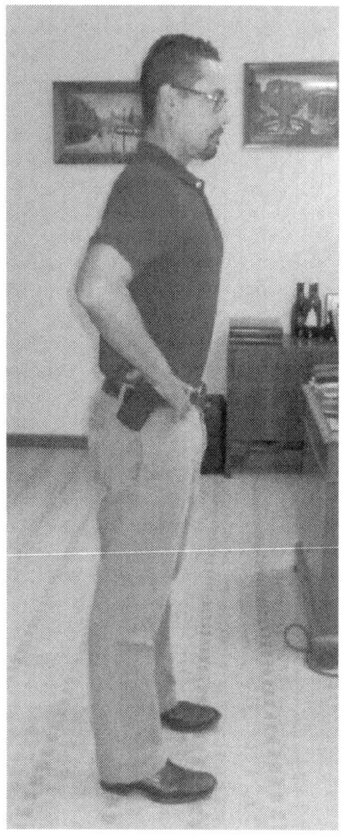

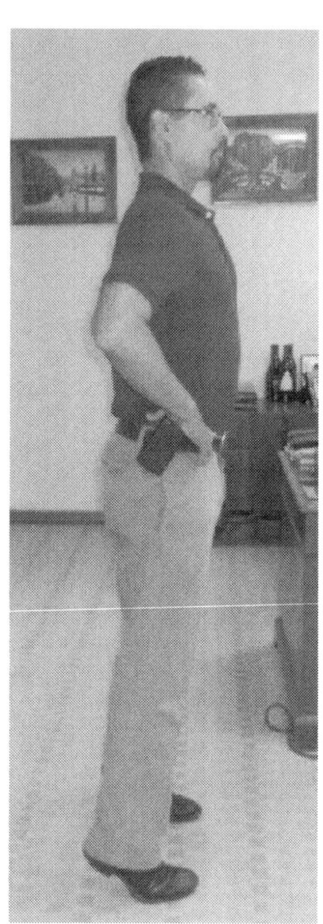

Calf Raises

13. Hamstring Curl with Band: Secure both ends of the band low to the ground on a stationary object. Wrap the band around the back of your right foot or ankle then stand facing the object. Pull the right heel up towards the right buttocks then return to original position. Repeat for 30 seconds then switch legs.

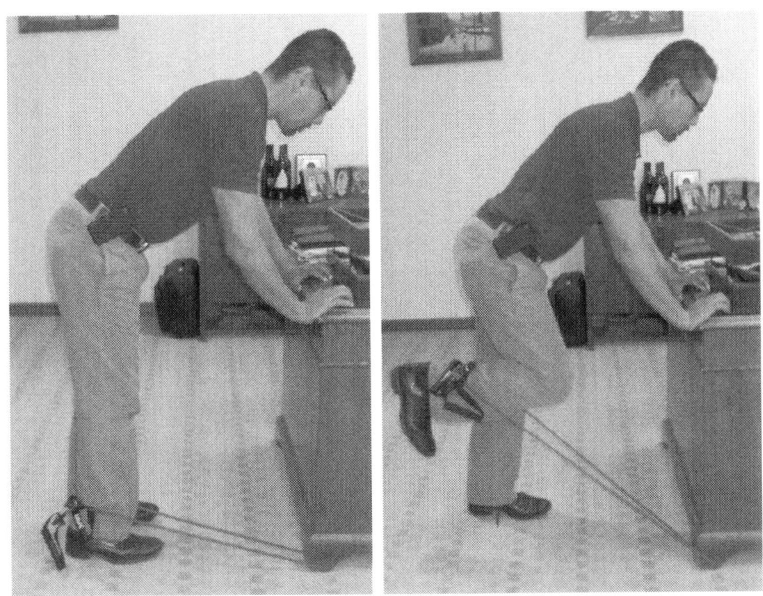

Hamstring Curl with Band

14. Knee Extensions with Band: Secure both ends of the band low to the ground on a stationary object. Wrap the band around your ankle and foot then sit facing away from the stationary object. Slowly extend your knee then return to the original position. Repeat for 30 seconds then switch legs.

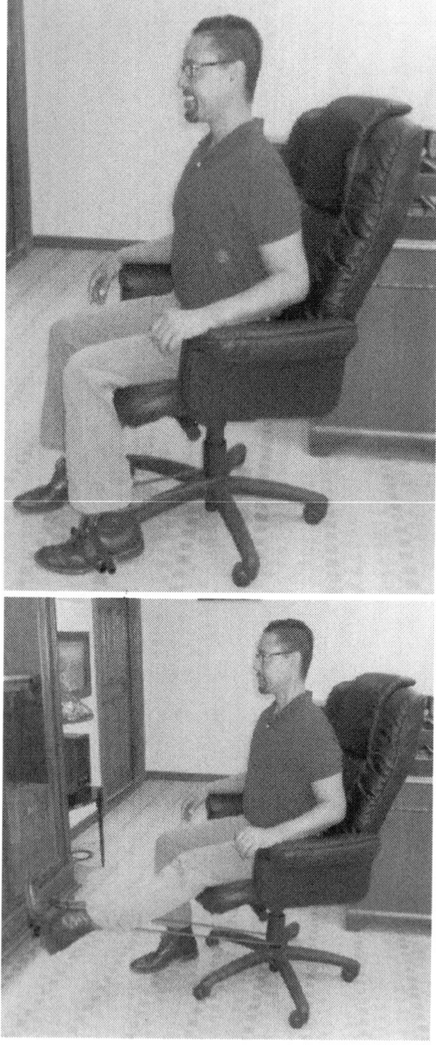

Knee Extensions with Band

15. Side Lunges: Begin in a standing position with feet hip distance apart. Step with the right foot to the right about 12-18 inches. Keep the left knee straight and bend the right knee, leaning out towards your right foot until you feel a gentle stretch on the inside of your left leg. Repeat for 30 seconds then switch sides.

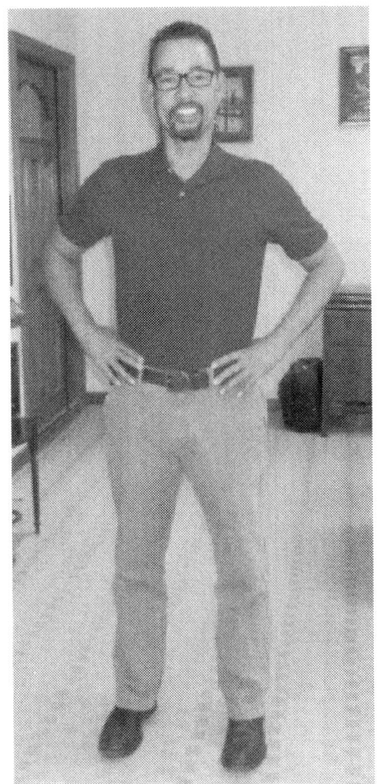

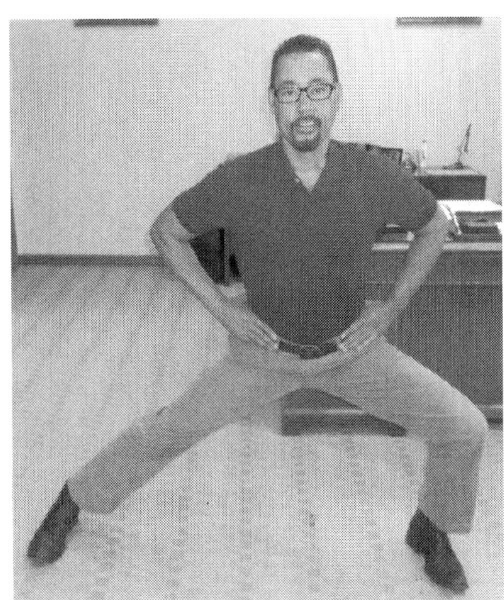

Side Lunges

16. Ball Squeezes: From a seated position place an exercise ball between your lower legs. Lift the ball off the ground and squeeze firmly holding the ball off the ground and squeezing for one minute.

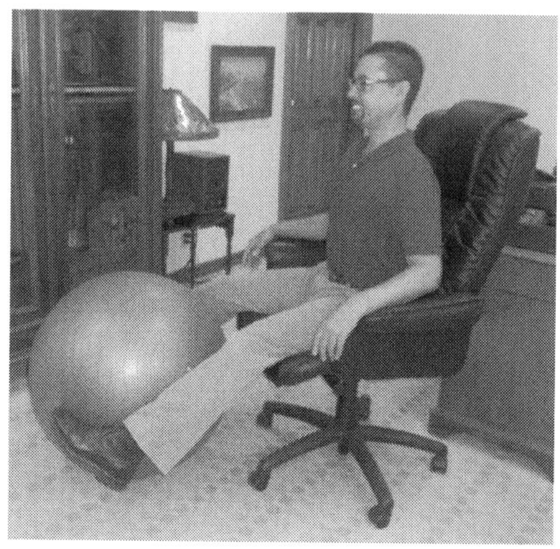

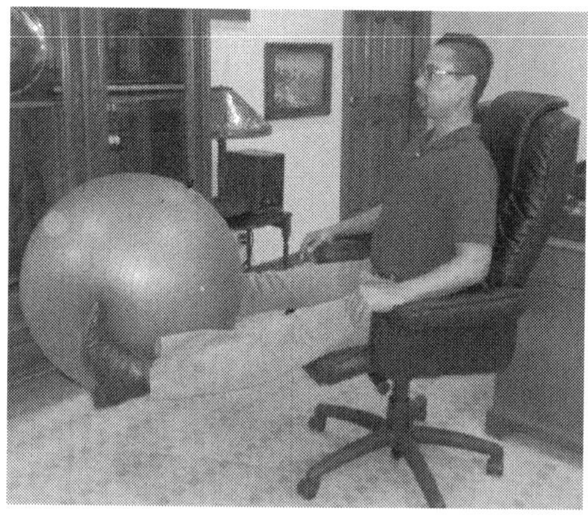

Ball Squeezes

17. Empty Step: Stand with your feet hip distance apart. Shift all of your weight onto your left foot and slowly lift your right foot off the ground. Bring your knee up slowly until it is even with your hip. Extend your right foot and bend your left knee, touching the toe of your right foot on the floor about 12 inches in front of you, putting no weight on the right foot (as if you were testing the temperature of the water in a lake you were thinking of swimming in). Lift the knee back up to hip level then return to your starting position. Repeat for 30 seconds balancing on the one leg the entire time. Switch legs.

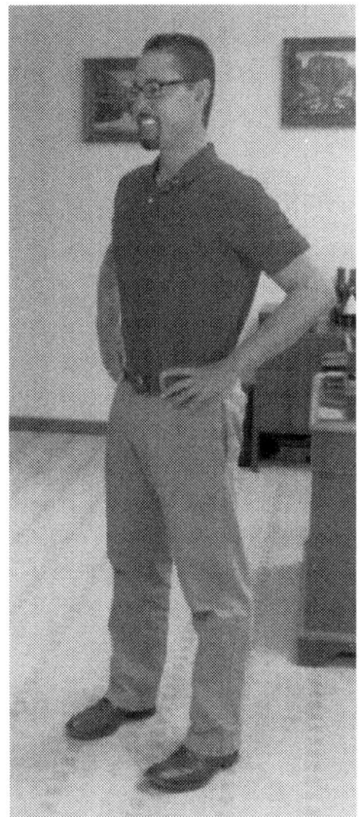

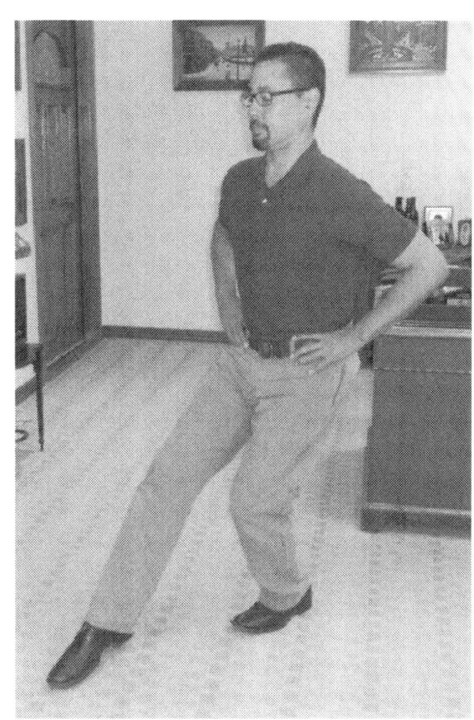

Empty Step

18. Wu Chi Stance: Stand with your feet slightly wider than hip distance apart. Bend your knees slightly (the deeper you bend your knees the more challenging this exercise becomes). Now tuck your tail bone under the spine, lengthening the lower back. Let your arms dangle at your sides. Roll your shoulders gently open and relax the chest. Allow your head to float off your shoulders. Hold for one minute.

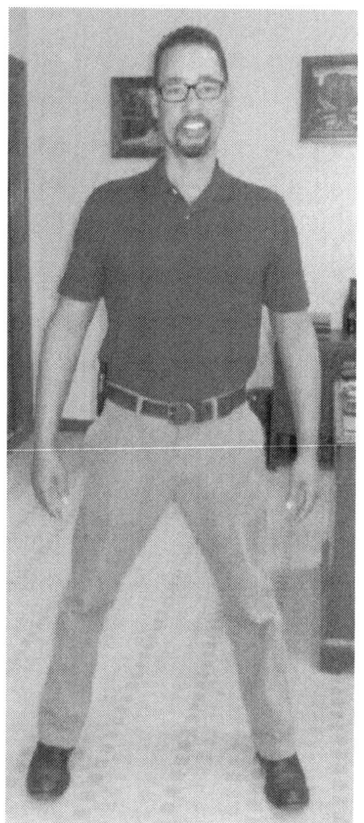

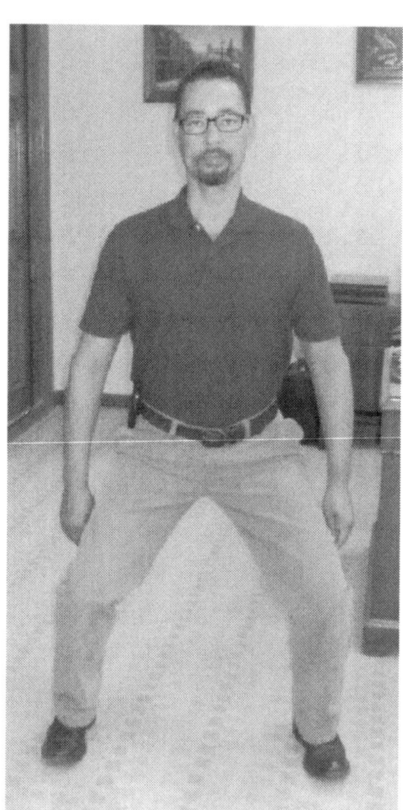

Wu Chi Stance

19. Dog Wags His Tail: From Wu Chi Stance, bring your hands down to the fronts of your thighs and rest them there. Bend your knees a little deeper, but be sure to keep the tail bone tucked under the spine, lower back long. Now slowly shift all of your weight over to your right foot and pause there for a moment (for more of a challenge, lift your left heel off the ground with only the toe touching).Then with both feet firmly on the ground again shift your weight over to your left foot and pause for a moment (you can lift the right heel if you wish). Go back and forth between the two feet for one minute.

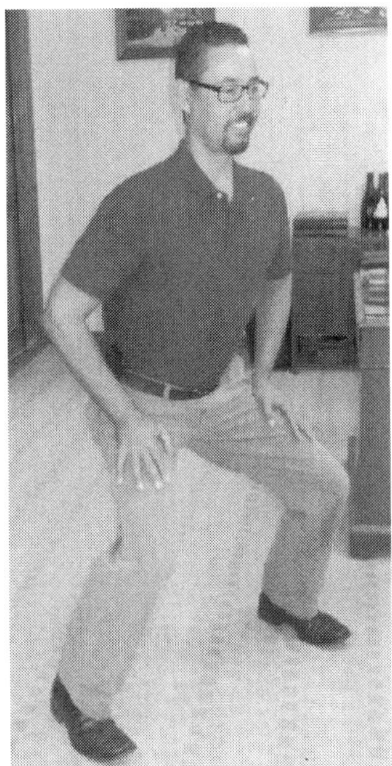

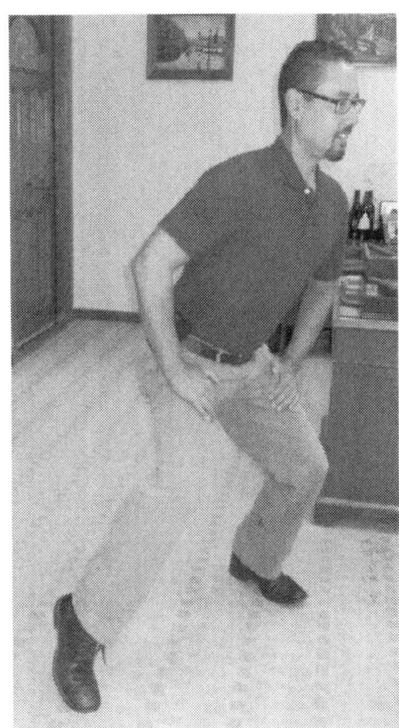

Dog Wags His Tail

20. Sumo Step: Stand with legs twice hip width apart. Drop the buttocks down six to 10 inches bringing you into a wide legged squat position (the deeper the squat the more challenging this becomes). Shift your weight over to your right foot and slowly lift your left foot off the ground 1 to 8 inches. Hold for a count of 5 then slowly lower the left foot back to the ground. Repeat on the opposite side. Continue for one minute.

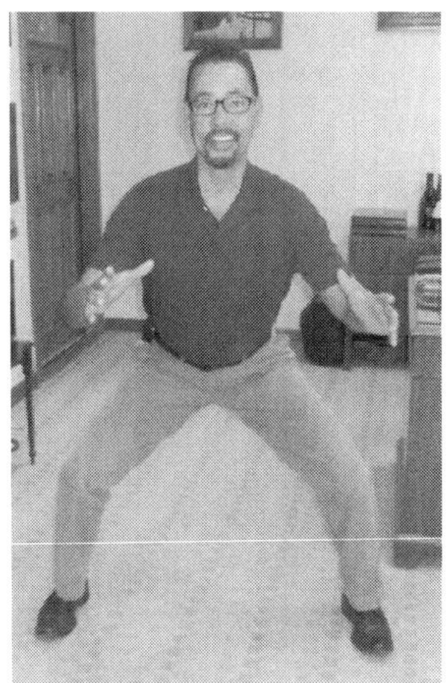
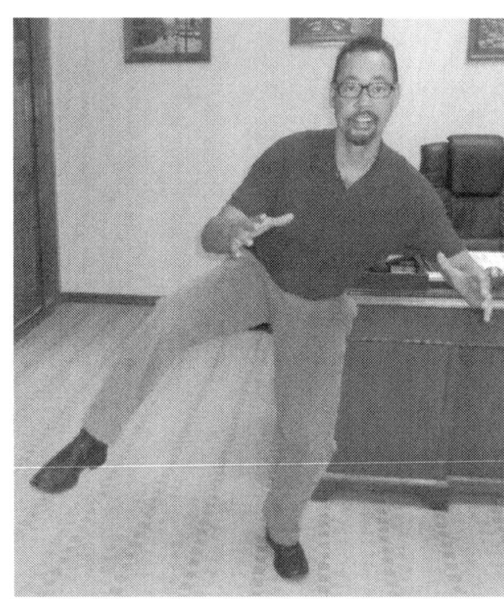

Sumo Step

21. Godzilla Walk: Wrap the band around both legs and tie it securely. Spread the legs as wide as possible then step forward with the right foot keeping the band taught. Then step forward with the left foot keeping the band taught. After that step back with the right foot keeping the band taught then step back with the left foot. Continue stepping forward and back keeping the band taught for one minute.

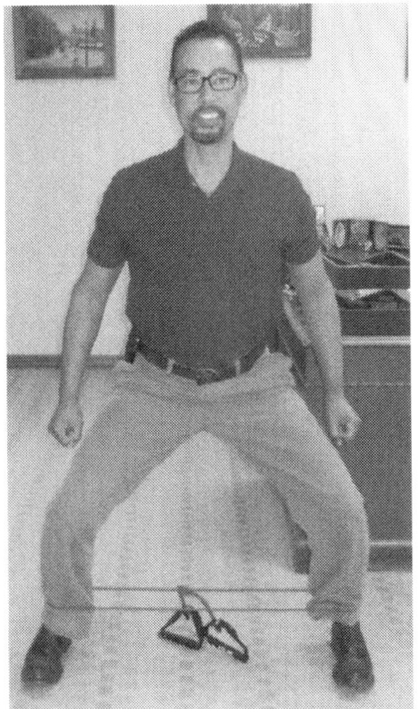

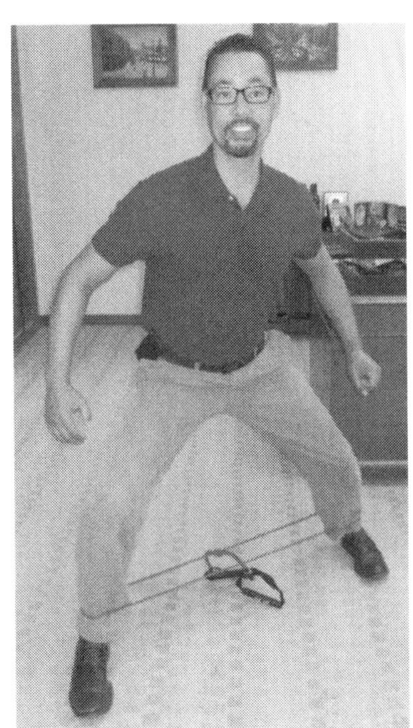

Godzilla Walk

22. Ball Hamstring Curls (double leg): Sitting in a chair place both feet on an exercise ball (your legs should be fully extended). Press your heels firmly down into the ball then pull the ball towards you trying to keep the ball moving in a straight line and pushing down hard into the ball with your heels. Press the legs away returning the ball to its original position. Repeat for one minute.

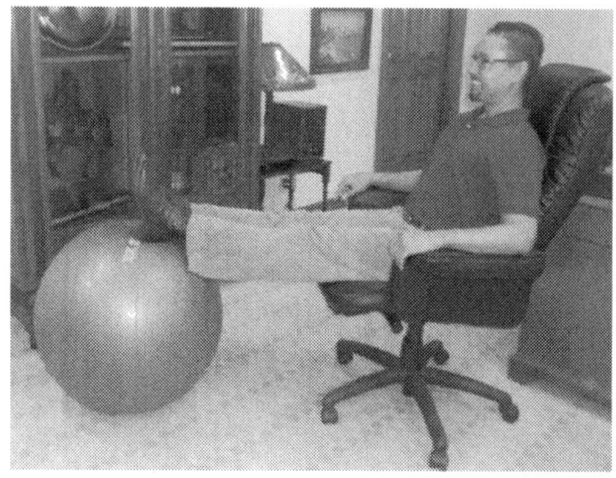

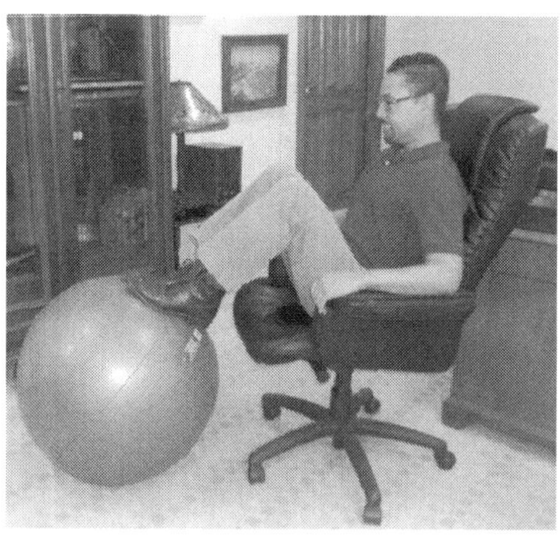

Ball Hamstring Curls (double leg)

23. Step Lunge: Stand with your feet slightly wider than hip distance apart. Place both hands on your hips. Step forward with your right foot approximately 18 to 24 inches. Bend your left knee and slowly kneel until the left knee touches or almost touches the floor. Be sure to keep the torso upright and the spine long. Keeping your feet where they are, slowly stand. Step back into original position and repeat with opposite leg. Alternate between legs for one minute.

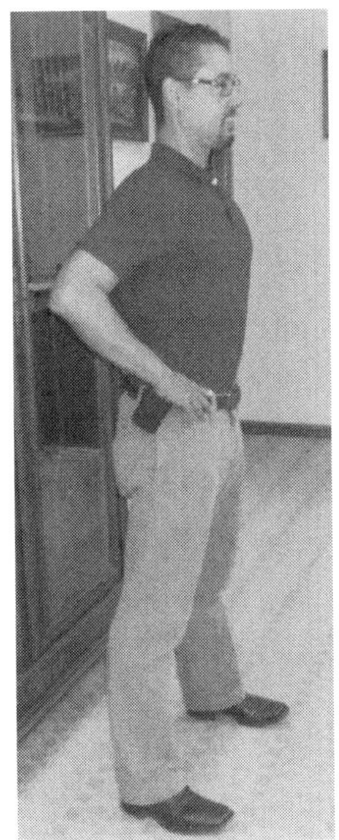

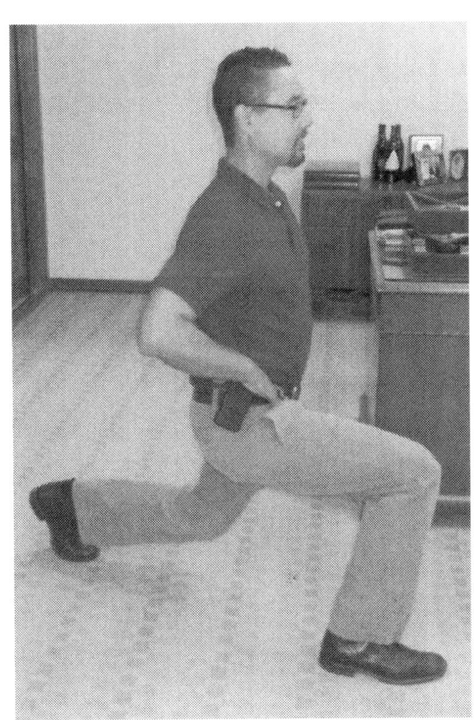

Step Lunge

24. Toe Point with Band: Attach both ends of the band to a stationary object near the ground. Loop the band around your ankle and face away from the object the band is attached to while keeping the band taught. Slowly lift your foot off the floor and point your toe at the ground and slide the foot forward, then return to the original position repeat for 30 seconds, then switch legs and repeat.

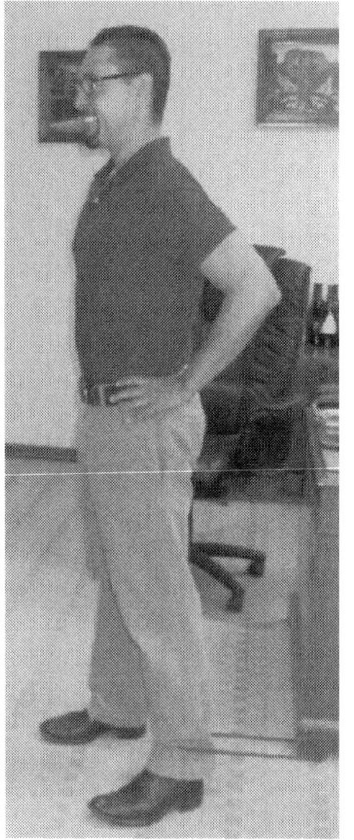

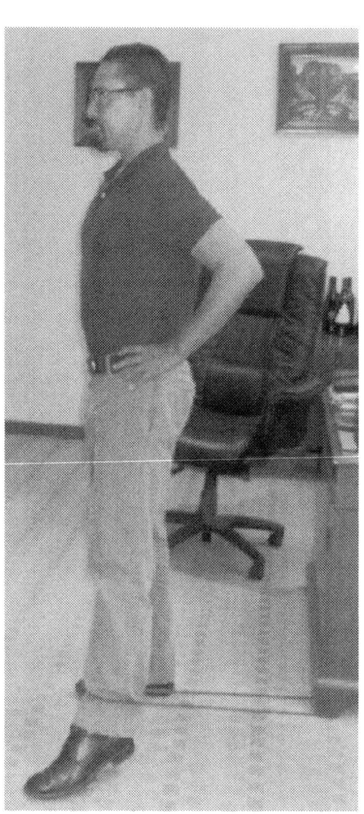

Toe Point with Band

25. Plie Squat: Stand with your hands on your hips. Spread your legs so they are slightly wider than hip distance apart with toes pointed outward at a 45-degree angle from the mid-line of the body. Bend your knees as you drop your buttocks down towards the floor as if you were going to sit in a chair, but be sure to keep your torso as upright as possible. Then return to the starting position. Repeat for one minute.

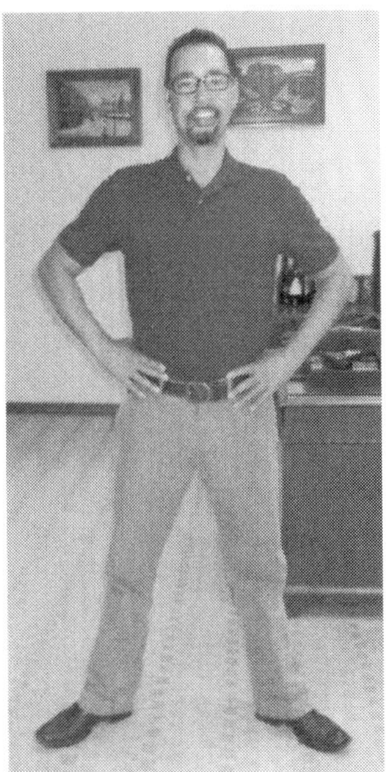

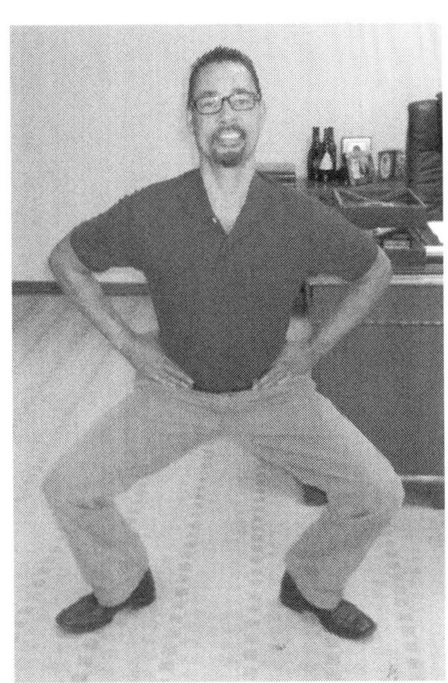

Plie Squat

11
The Lower Body Strength Program

I have created a sample three day lower body strength training program for the office. This program was designed for people who only want to work on lower body strength. Each of the exercises listed below should be done for exactly one minute. If you decide to do all five exercises each hour, you should be back to work after no more than five minutes. (If you are pressed for time in any given hour, just do 2 or 3 of the exercises and get back to work!)

Day 1

9:45

- Chair squats
- Tush Tightener
- Side Beats
- Calf Raises
- Ball Hamstring Curls (single leg)

10:45

- Wall Squats
- Crossovers
- Single Leg Rolling Lunges
- Knee Extension with Band
- Curtsy Raise

11:45

- The Kick

- Wide Leg Squat
- Toe Point with Band
- Dog Wags his Tail
- Step Lunge

1:45

- Empty Step
- Wu Chi Stance
- Ball Squeezes
- Godzilla Walk
- Ball Hamstring Curls (double leg)

2:45

- Touch Down
- Curtsy Raise
- Empty Step
- Calf Raises
- Ball Squeezes

Day 2

10:45

- Step Lunge
- Dog Wags his Tail
- Plie Squat
- Single Leg Rolling Lunges
- Ball Squeezes

11:45

- Knee Extension with Band
- Empty Step
- Crossover
- Godzilla Walk

- Ball Hamstring Curls (single leg)

1:45

- Single Leg Rolling Lunges
- The Kick
- Side Lunge
- Wu Chi Stance
- Sumo Step

2:45

- Ball Hamstring Curls (double leg)
- Chair Squats
- Tush Tightener
- Toe Point with Band
- Curtsy Raise

3:45

- Wall Squats
- Side Beats
- Touch Down
- Ball Squeezes
- Single Leg Rolling Lunges

Day 3

9:45

- Touch Down
- Empty Step
- The Kick
- Wall Squat
- Step Lunge

10:45

- Side Lunges
- Curtsy Raises

- Godzilla Walk
- Side Beats
- Sumo Step

11:45

- Crossovers
- Ball Squeezes
- Plie Squat
- Wu Chi Stance
- Toe point with Band

1:45

- Chair Squats
- Knee Extensions with Band
- Ball Hamstring Curls (single leg)
- Tush Tightener
- Ball Hamstring Curls (double leg)

2:45

- Single Leg Rolling Lunges
- Empty Step
- Dog Wags his Tail
- Calf Raises
- Wide Leg Squat

3-day Upper & Lower Body Program

This program is for people who would like to do a full body workout

3-day program
Day 1

9:45

- Touch Down
- Empty Step
- The Kick
- Wall Squat
- Step Lunge

10:45

- Scaption
- Concentration Curls
- Push Up
- Reverse Fly
- Wood Chop

11:45

- Knee Extension with Band
- Ball Squeezes
- Crossover
- Godzilla Walk
- Ball Hamstring Curls (single leg)

1:45

- Shoulder Presses
- Reverse Curls
- Single Arm Chest Fly
- Bent Over Row
- The Hug

2:45

- Chair Squats
- Curtsy Raise
- Single Leg Rolling Lunges
- Calf Raises
- Plie Squat

Day 2

10:45

- Front Raises
- Concentration Curls
- Wide Arm Push Up
- Shrug
- Wood Chop

11:45

- Side Lunges
- Curtsy Raises
- Godzilla Walk
- Side Beats
- Sumo Step

1:45

- Lateral Raises
- Reverse Curls
- Chest Fly
- Seated Row
- Scaption

2:45

- Single Leg Rolling Lunges
- Empty Step
- Dog Wags his Tail

- Calf Raises
- Wide Leg Squat

3:45

- Wall Squats
- Side Beats
- Touch Down
- Ball Squeezes
- Single Leg Rolling Lunges
-

Day 3

9:45

- Chair Squats
- Tush Tightener
- Side Beats
- Calf Raises
- Ball Hamstring Curls (single leg)

10:45

- Lateral Raises
- Biceps Curls
- Standing Chest Press
- Seated Row
- Shrug

11:45

- Crossovers
- Ball Squeezes
- Plie Squat
- Wu Chi Stance
- Toe Point with Band

1:45

- Front Punch
- Hammer Curls
- Wide Arm Push Up
- Bent Over Row (single handed)
- Wing Curl (single handed)

2:45

- Ball Hamstring Curls (double leg)
- Chair Squat
- Tush Tightener
- Toe Point with Band
- Curtsy Raise

12
Your Back, Why it Probably Hurts, and My Back Story

If you suffer from back pain, don't feel like the Lone Ranger. Eighty percent of all people in the western industrialized societies will experience some form of back pain in their lifetime (we will get into more statistics later). In fact I bring my own baggage and insights to this subject. I lettered in four sports each year of high school, then went on to play football for Saginaw Valley State University. It was both heaven and hell. Playing college football had always been my dream. It enforced my sense of self-worth, since I knew people back home were following my athletic career. But college football put intense importance on winning: losing seasons could cost staff members their jobs and the athletes felt the pressure. As a wide receiver, spectacular catches were expected of me-so I sacrificed my body to the defensive backs during each practice, hoping for a place in the starting lineup.

During the first game in my sophomore year, I was sprinting across the field for a reception when another player slammed his helmeted head like a battering ram into the center of my lower back. After the hit I got up feeling stiff, but played the rest of the game. On the bus trip home my back hurt, but that wasn't unusual. Later in my dorm room, my back muscles began to spasm. In an attempt to relax the muscles, I got down on the floor to stretch. I felt something tear and heard a loud crack, *and everything from my chest down went dead.* I lay there in the dark on the floor. No feeling, no movement. Nothing. I convinced myself that I wasn't scared: a few weeks earlier, a "stinger," or pinched nerve in my neck had left one arm numb and useless for several hours. I told myself that this was the same thing.

I woke up my roommate, who called the trainers. Bleary-eyed, they arrived at my room and checked my reflexes-but found none. They exchanged nervous glances as one of them called an ambulance. After hours of X-rays and a battery of other tests, a doctor came to my bedside.

"I have some bad news," he began.

With the arrogance of youth, I finished his sentence inside my head: *You're out for the season, son.* I prepared myself, knowing I should take it like a man. How would I deal with being on the sidelines for an entire season? What would my coach say? The doctor's next words made those questions seem trivial.

"You've crushed two disks and cracked the vertebrae in several pieces in between. Pieces of the vertebrae have shifted into the spinal cord, putting pressure on it. There's a great deal of swelling. You may walk again in an hour. You may never walk again. We honestly don't know."

The rest of the doctor's speech fell on deaf ears. I didn't know what to say or what to do. Too numb to make a decision, I cried myself to sleep that night, alone in a hospital room hundreds of miles from home. The next few days were a waiting game to see if the swelling would go down so the doctors could determine the extent of the damage to my spine cord. I had never been so devastated; just one week earlier I had made a spectacular catch in front of hundreds of screaming fans. Now I couldn't even move my legs. My hospital roommate was a young quadriplegic man, the victim of a motorcycle accident five years before. He was in the hospital because his caregiver had placed him in too-hot bathwater; neither of them had realized until his skin turned bright red and began to blister. I imagined myself in his place. One night as we lay talking in the glow from the television screen, he told me not to give up hope.

"With hard work, you can make progress." With extreme effort he lifted his hand two inches off the bed then almost imperceptibly wiggled his fingers. He smiled and dropped his hand to the bed with a tired sigh.

"I worked three years to do that," he said proudly. Then, exhausted, he fell asleep.

Christ, I thought to myself, *the poor guy can't even lift his hand to wipe his own brow*. Then I realized my plight wasn't much better. Later, I called my best buddy at the college and asked him to smuggle in a pint of Southern Comfort. I drank and cried myself to sleep that night. After a battery of tests my doctors said that there didn't seem to be any major spinal cord damage but there was a lot of swelling in and around the spine so they prescribed anti inflammatory and pain medication. I couldn't move my legs and was relegated to a wheelchair. I would lie on ice beds, did physical therapy and was put in traction (weights tied to your feet and neck to stretch the spine) for hours a day but saw no improvement. I spent almost a month in the hospital but there was no change in my condition and finally they sent me home.

"Maybe the swelling will go down on its own over time" they told me, "try to be patient and we will see what happens over the course of the next few months."

But nine months later there still was no change in my condition. Finally my mother interceded and convinced me to go and have the surgery. Surgeons removed the two damaged disks and fragments of debris, then fused the vertebrae in what at the time was a new "experimental" procedure. For two days nothing happened. On the third morning, I awoke to searing pain shooting down both of my legs. It hurt like hell, but the tears rolling down my cheeks were from joy, not pain. Unable to speak, I watched as my toes barely moved up and down at my bidding.

I had been given a second chance to walk, and I could hardly wait to start. But the muscles in my midsection and legs had atrophied severely during their nine month hiatus. My body weight had dropped from a hearty 185 pounds to a scrawny 140 and my legs looked like withered sticks. After the surgery I began physical therapy with a woman they called the "Hippy Lady." At first the Hippy Lady was nice, she was helpful and encouraging, but progress was painfully slow. The more I worked with her the more she began to tick me off. Her cheerfulness grated on me, her encouragement only made me want to do the opposite of whatever she said. Frustrated and angry at the world, I lashed out at her.

"This crap is useless--just a big waste of time" I screamed." I've been doing this therapy for over a year and I'm still in that wheelchair, what good are you?"

Each session was worse than the last as I became more and more belligerent and I was drinking more as well--sometimes even showing up to therapy drunk. Finally she took me aside.

"Look," she said. "I've had just about enough. Our sessions are starting to take on a theme and that theme is you complaining more and giving less effort. If you don't want to walk that's fine with me! I have lots of people who want to get better and I don't have time to screw around with someone who's giving up. So why don't you just and crawl into that bottle of booze you love so much and do us all a favor and stop wasting my time." Now that she had my attention she followed up with:

"You're probably right about one thing, physical therapy probably isn't helping you, but I know something that will." Now she really had my attention. She looked around as if to make sure no one was listening, then continued.

"There is an ancient technique that predates history that is incredibly powerful; so powerful that they have banned me from teaching it here. This technique not only transforms your body but awakens the powers beyond your imagination hidden deep inside your mind. Now this was 1981 and I was 20 years old and I had seen Star Wars and The Empire Strikes Back and all I could think was "Luke, use the force." So now I was all ears. She looked around again and lowered her voice:

"If they even knew I was talking with you about this I would probably get fired. But if you're interested in *really* changing your life, the physical therapy office closes at 5:00 p.m. Come down at 5:30. *No one can know we're doing this, do you understand!"* I nodded my head.

"I mean this," she said, "Before you come down here, think about it long and hard because if you do decide to come down, it won't be easy and you will have to do exactly what I tell you to do but it will change your life!" She looked at me with cold hard eyes, "5:30. At 5:31, I'm gone." She stated flatly.

Looking back at this exchange 30 years later I'm pretty sure she played me. Don't get me wrong. What she said that day was absolutely true; the ancient technique she was talking about was yoga and it *did* change my life. It did give me powers beyond my 20 year-old imagination and it was instrumental in helping me recover but she played me nonetheless. In the time we had worked together she had sized me up and then pushed all the right buttons to get me to do what she knew I needed to do to recover. The woman was brilliant!

Over the next couple of months I snuck down to the physical therapy offices every night. She not only taught me yoga but also the exercises of Joseph Pilates as well as other things like meditation, visualization, and the critical connection between the body and the mind. I learned about meditation, mantras, creative visualization, breathing techniques and concentration meditations. I developed a healthy back routine that combined physical therapy exercises with yoga and pilates that helped keep my back, core and associated muscle groups strong yet supple and I did those exercises regularly. Not only did I fully regain the use of my legs but I went on to become a yoga instructor, Pilates instructor, personal trainer and wellness expert. Now this would be the perfect place to write "and he lived happily ever after," but that's not really the whole story.

Fast forward almost thirty years and I'm working at a top health spa in California teaching four to six hours of exercise classes a day. It's been several years since I've had the time or energy to do my little back health routine but I figure I'm exercising every day, so I don't need no stinkin' back health routine. One day after leading a cross-fit style class I noticed that my right hamstring felt tight. In all honesty I didn't give it much thought, because in my line of work a little stiffness and soreness comes with the territory. But over the course of the next few weeks the hamstring just got worse, going from tight to painful. Finally I went to the doctor who took an x ray and declared I had an inflamed tendon, put me on anti inflammatory meds and sent me off to physical therapy. But after just a couple of weeks at the PT my therapist pulled me aside and said,

"There's something not right about this. The doctor says the inflammation is in the front of the hip but your pain is in the back of your leg,"

He went on to say that as we had been working together that he had noticed weakness in my right leg that seemed to be getting worse. He sent me back to the doctor for an MRI of my low back and hip joint. What the MRI revealed shocked me. The neurologist said that the fusion that was done back in the 80s had "failed" and I had significant arthritis and bone spurs and that the vertebra that were supposed to be fused were moving around freely. Add to that a couple of seriously herniated disks, and my back was, well….a train wreck.

To my surprise he did not recommend surgery; he said that the outcomes from back surgery aren't very good and it should be the last thing to consider after we had tried everything else and nothing had worked. So he sent me back to the physical therapist. The only problem was I was still working, teaching four to six hours of exercise classes five days a week. Over the next few weeks my right leg got weaker and I began to experience more and more pain that shot down the leg. What I became aware of is just doing any kind of exercise isn't enough to keep your back healthy and over-training can be as bad for your back and overall health as not training enough. Finally one day while heading down the flight of stairs to my basement office, my right leg buckled under me and I took a fall down the steps. It was then I realized it was time to stop working that job.

Over the next 6 months things just got worse until I was using a cane to walk. Finally I decided to go back to my original healthy back routine (which includes many of the 25 exercises in this book) and do it regularly (at least 4 days a week).This simple change made all the difference. Slowly I improved. My right leg grew stronger, the pain slowly subsided and I started to move back into a space where I felt normal again. I walk 4-8 miles a day and do my exercises faithfully. Life is good again.

I want to stress that each of us are different and what works for me may not work for you, so it's important to experiment and create your own healthy back routine, but the 25 exercises in this book are a great place to start and creating a routine that you can do at work means never having to say "I don't have time to exercise." It also means that you will be able to regularly get out of the thing that is probably the worst enemy of your back…your office chair. Fitting in a few minutes of movement each hour is easy and will help not only your back but your overall health and believe it or not actually benefit your employer as well (more about that later).

Keep in mind these exercises are meant to be done when you are not in spasm or severe pain. If you are experiencing pain you should always contact a medical professional for a diagnosis and the appropriate treatment for you. As you read further into this book you will see that the right kind of regular exercise will make your back strong, supple and reduce and maybe even eliminate the amount of pain you experience, so let's get you started down the road to a healthier back!

13
"But Why?"

When I was growing up I was one of those kids that whenever you asked me to do something the first thing out of my mouth was "why?" Why was a very important question for me and the answer I got often determined how much time, energy, effort went into what you asked me to do or for that matter if it got done at all. Let me give you an example. In my house Saturday night was steak night, every Saturday we had steak, a baked potato with butter, sour cream and chives as well as a vegetable. Now I loved the steak and potato but the vegetable…not so much. This is how it went almost every Saturday. My mom would hand out plates loaded with food to the family. I would say grace then dig into my steak like a ravenous grizzly bear. My mother would look at me and say "Kent, eat your vegetables" to which I would reply "why?" Her three standard answers were "because I put a lot of work into making those," or "they're good for you" or "because I said so."

None of these answers did much to motivate me, so I would sneak as much of my vegetables to the dog as he would eat and what he turned his nose up to, I snuck into my pockets so later that evening I could toss the evidence out my bedroom window. That was pretty much the Saturday night routine. Then one night my mom handed me a plate with a new vegetable I had never seen before. She told me they were Brussels Sprouts. She said,

"Eat your Brussels Sprouts," and when I said "Why?" Mom threw me a curve ball. "They'll help you grow big muscles," she said.

This was new and very interesting to me because I was a skinny little kid and I didn't have any muscles…but I wanted them.

"How do they do that?" I asked suspiciously.

"The vitamins and minerals in the Brussels Sprouts work with the steak to help your body grow big muscles," she explained. And then she hit me with the real zinger:

"I read it in Woman's Day Magazine."

Holy crap! I thought. If they wrote it in Woman's Day it had to be true! I looked down at the Brussels Sprouts, and man, were they green! I couldn't think of anything I liked that was green. I sniffed them; they smelled bad, bitter with a hint of rotten egg. I cut one in half and plopped it in my mouth. It was awful! It tasted like how I imagined my underwear would taste after wearing them for a week straight. I gagged and got ready to spit the disgusting thing back onto my plate. But before I did I looked down at my arms and they looked like twigs sticking out of my T shirt. I looked at my legs. My dad often teased that he had seen bigger legs on birds. Rather than spit out the mouthful of Brussels Sprouts, I quickly chewed it up and swallowed it, washing the taste out of my mouth with a big gulp of ice cold milk. It wasn't easy but by the end of dinner I had polished off all of them. My mom smiled at me, tousled my hair and as she cleared the table said

"If you keep that up, the dog's gonna waste away."

My point here is that for many people, *why* we're doing something can be a very powerful motivator for actually getting it done. If you're one of those people, then this chapter is for you. In this chapter I will give you all the reasons you should want a healthy back. If you're one of those people that simply wants to know *what* to do and statistics and facts are just going to bore you and delay you in getting started, then just skip this chapter and move on!

So who exactly gets back pain? The answer to that question is *almost everyone*. Consider these facts:

- It is estimated that back pain effects over 31 million Americans and is the number one cause of activity limitation in young adults
- Within a given year, up to 50% of U.S. adults suffer from back pain
- Americans spend at least $50 billion each year on low back pain and it is the second most common neurological ailment in the United States
- Low back pain is the second most frequent reason for visits to the physician
- 80% of people over the age of 30 will experience back problems at some point in their lives. 30% of those will have recurring problems
- Each year, there are approximately 916,000 spinal surgeries performed in the U.S. alone
- Back pain accounts for almost one fourth of all occupational injuries and illnesses
- In the United States, back surgery rates increase almost proportionally with the supply of orthopedic and neurosurgeons

More fun facts about back pain from our friends at the National Institute of Musculoskeletal and Skin Diseases:

- Back pain is more common among older adults.
- Lack of fitness can cause back pain people who are not very fit suffer more from back pain.
- Inherited diseases such as disc diseases which can cause back pain.
- Being overweight can also cause back pain.
- Other kind of diseases can also cause back pain such as cancer and arthritis.
- Work related back pain. Some kinds of work may require you to end or twist the back which can cause pain.
- Smoking can also delay the cure of back pain.

- Racial factors can also be a cause of back pain. Black women often suffer from displacement of lower spine compared to white women.
- According to estimates 4 out of 5 adults will experience back pain in their lives.
- Back pain is very common health problem. In 2000 almost half of the UK adult population (49%) complained about back pain which lasted for about 24 hours sometime during that year.
- Simple measures can be taken up to prevent back pain.
- First aid help prevents the aggravation of the back pain.
- It is important to remain active even if one has back pain.
- In most cases back pain is not very serious.
- Back pain can start among school children and peak among adults between the ages of 35 to 55 years.
- Heavy physical work, lifting heavy objects and sitting straight for long hours can cause back pain.
- Psychosocial factors such stress, anxiety, depression, mental stress and lack of job satisfaction can also cause back pain.
- Nearly 90% of the people with back pain will recover within 6 weeks.

Why Sitting at Your Desk is so bad for Your Back

Back pain is not a life-threatening disease, but having chronic back pain can make life pretty unbearable. Take it from a guy who broke his back at the tender age of 19, was a paraplegic for a year, and has dealt with back pain ever since. The chair you're sitting in right now probably isn't helping you much if you suffer from back pain, even if it is super expensive and says it's ergonomically correct.

"Short of sitting on a spike, you can't do much worse than a standard office chair," says Dr. Galen Cranz, a professor of environmental design at the University of California at Berkeley. The problem is that the spine simply wasn't designed to stay in the seated position for long periods of time. For the most part, the slight S shape of the spine serves us well. "If you think about a heavy weight on a C or S, which is going to collapse more easily? The C," she says. But when you sit, the lower portion of the back known as the lumbar spine has its curve collapse, turning the spine's natural S-shape into a C, hampering the core musculature that support the body. The body ends up slouching and the muscles through the ribcage and all of the postural muscles lose their strength and cease to function properly from lack of use, leaving you out of balance and in a poor spinal position, and *voilà*: back pain.

This, in turn, causes problems with other parts of the body. "When you're standing, you're bearing weight through the hips, knees, and ankles," says Dr. Andrew C. Hecht, co-chief of spinal surgery at Mount Sinai Medical Center. "When you're sitting, you're bearing all that weight through the pelvis and spine, and it puts the highest pressure on your back discs. Looking at MRIs, even sitting with perfect posture causes serious pressure on your back."

My good friend Dr. Logan Osland, a chiropractor in Ventura, California sees patients every day that are in severe pain because of sitting for most of their day. "As a chiropractor I talk to people on a daily basis about how bad it is to sit all the time," Dr. Osland says. "From just a mechanical perspective, our core and gluteal musculature activity volume decreases dramatically. Our anterior hip musculature becomes tight from being in a constant shortened position. As a result our low backs have to take on more responsibility for movement, which eventually causes injury." But it isn't just our lower back that is affected by long bouts of sitting.

According to Dr. Osland, sitting can also have negative repercussions on the neck, shoulders, and mid-back. "The problem for these areas is everything is out in front of us. Our back is stabilized, causing vertebrae to become immobile; the shoulder blades move out wider; arms internally rotate; neck becomes straight and the head moves forward." In chiropractic terms this is referred to as FHP, or forward head posture. FHP can lead to headaches, neck pain, and upper-extremity nerve entrapment syndromes (like carpal tunnel and cubital tunnel). According to Dr. Osland, "low back pain is the second leading cause of missed work days, second only to the common cold." What's obvious here is that sitting is not good for spinal alignment, and since the spine houses the spinal cord which sends all the messages from the brain to the rest of the body, spinal alignment is pretty darned important. The only way to relieve the pressures on the spine caused by sitting is to get up and move. This forces the postural muscles to activate, allows blood to flow through the spinal region, and gets us back to moving the way that nature intended.

Another colleague, Breena Maggio, Restorative Exercise Specialist and owner of "The Body Education Alignment Center for Health" in Ventura, California puts it this way:"Many people don't realize that the detriment of sitting is not just in the not moving, but in these two primary things: 1) the change to the resting length of the muscles that happens when the body is in a static position for 8-16 hours per day, every day and 2) the change to the geometry of your blood vessels from maintaining this static position for hours on end, which affects how your blood flows through your blood vessels. Most people also don't realize just how many hours per day then spend in a sitting position of hip and knee flexion (think work, driving, exercise machines, bikes, couches, mealtimes)- count them, you'll be surprised." Maggio goes on to say,

"First, to address the change in resting length of the muscles: Your body (every single system, tissue and cell) works best, when it is aligned as nature intended. We are designed to be moving creatures, not static creatures, and movement is different from exercise. To maintain this optimal alignment requires all of your muscles. That's ALL of them, not just the 12 or so major muscles you work at the gym, to be at their correct length."

This means that the little postural and stabilizer muscles are just as important as the big muscles.

"When your body is in one position for many hours per day, this is your training program. Your hamstrings, calves, and hip flexors are in a chronically shortened position and you are training them to maintain this shortened position. The flip side of this is that to be able to stand up in alignment and walk optimally, you need your hamstrings, calves, and hip flexors to be at their optimal length."

She continues,

"Muscles that are too short are muscles that have very little innervation. And muscles that are lowly innervated use less energy and have less space to carry blood, which means higher blood pressure overall in your cardiovascular system. It also means, if you have great quantities of muscle that you are not able to use because the muscles are not innervated, you have a lower basal metabolic rate (metabolism) than you should have. Metabolic Syndrome anyone? Diabetes? Obesity? It really is amazing, but it's true: Stretching alone (proper stretching) can be the best weight loss program you've ever tried."

"Second, the change in the geometry of your blood vessels is a bigger contributor- actually it's the major contributor- to the increased risk of death. The reason that sitting increases the risk of death is much simpler than the fat, cholesterol, and chemistry that we are trying to make it…it's about geometry. Your body's circulatory system is arranged in such a way to maximize optimal blood flow. When you add random twists and turns to your blood vessels, which you do with chronic sitting, you affect the flow of your blood. What actually is happening on the cellular level, is an increase in the number and frequency of "wall wounding". This is what causes plaques to form on the arterial walls. A blood cell bangs up against the blood vessel wall and creates a wound. This is the first stage of plaque accumulation. Allow this to keep happening over and over again, and you've got yourself some cardiovascular disease. Exercise doesn't affect the wall wound or the wounding itself. But you can change your blood vessel geometry for the good and stop the wounding just as easily as you bent it all up when you sat down."

"Stand up. When you stand up, you remove all the arbitrary bends and curves you created when you sat down. Understand that if you've been sitting for many hours, for many days, for many years, your muscles, and thus your bones and joints, are not yet ready to jump up and stand for 8 hours straight. You need to add the necessary stretching. Start with a simple calf stretch done using a half foam roller. Do this multiple times throughout the day. Heck, you're already standing, it's easy to stretch your calves at the same time. Actually, the best thing you can do for your body is to change positions frequently. You can sit when you need to. Stand for part of the time. Even squat. Yes, I said squat. Can you sit on the floor for part of your workday?"

"Unfortunately, despite what fitness and the media have been telling us for years, we cannot make up for not moving and undo the chronic sitting position we hold our bodies in for 8-16 hours per day, with a short bout of intense exercise. It's impossible. This is why, in the studies done on the deadly effects of sitting, those who exercised and those who did not, were at equal increased risk of death. Exercise does not undo the damage done by the change to the muscles length and the blood vessel geometry. Therefore, sitting on an exercise bike to do your work isn't going to undo it either. Also, since the only way to walk on a treadmill is to flex at the hip and put one leg out in front, this is not the solution to undoing all that sitting hip flexion either." Maggio concludes,

"Some of the changes you'll need to make are contrary to what you think you can do. But you're going to have to think a little differently about what is "normal" or what your coworkers will think if you want to save yourself from your maniacal killer chair."

Although this research is very much in its infancy, scientists and researchers all over the world are delving into the effects of sitting for extended periods of time on the human body and our overall health. As more of this research comes in, we will get a clearer picture of exactly how much we need to move to stay healthy and lower our risk of developing ailments like heart disease, diabetes, obesity and cancer. But what is clear even today is that our bodies were designed to be, and need to be, active on a regular basis, and for many of us our current lifestyle is not keeping up with those very basic needs. If you're a "the glass is half empty" kind of person, you might be thinking that this is just more bad news—just another group of scientists with the voice of doom and gloom predicting our early demise. But that's not the case at all. Our technology has lead us down a road that turned out to be a bit of a dead end health-wise, but we haven't traveled very far down that road, and getting back on the right track won't take much time.

The real message here is that the fix is an incredibly easy one. This simple fix will make you feel better and more energized. It will make you more productive, lengthen your life and lessen your pain, and you can accomplish all that by just standing up! And if you can do all that by just standing up, think of what you could accomplish if you did movements that improved your strength, balance, flexibility and energy. We aren't talking about hours of drudgery here. We're talking just minutes a day! I'm not sure how the news could get any better, unless of course it came in a pill--but nothing worth having is that easy. So now it is time to stand up for your health, literally! In a few chapters you will learn simple movements that can help you in many ways, but you have to be willing to take the first step.

14
Stress and Back Pain

Stress is a fact of life. Most of us live with a certain amount of stress every day. Much of that stress is caused by our jobs. Maybe it's that looming deadline, an unhappy boss or client no matter what the cause; stress can take a toll on our health. The thing that most of us don't understand is it's not the stress that messes with your health it's how you handle the stress. While many may be aware that un-controlled stress can lead to lowered immune function and can contribute to heart disease few are aware that stress can also lead to back pain. For the purpose of this book there are two kinds of stress; there is physical stress and emotional stress.

Physical stress happens when we ask the body to perform a task that is very difficult like lift a heavy object or run very fast for an extended period of time. This kind of stress can actually be good for your body. When you put a controlled amount of this kind of stress on the body it actually makes muscles stronger, the heart more efficient and increases lung capacity. But put too much physical stress on the body and it can lead to injury.

Emotional stress is different, with emotional stress the body isn't put under any direct duress, with this stress it's all in your head. What do I mean by emotional stress? Your boss walks into your work space and says "tomorrow's presentation had better be good, we lose the Harrison contract and it could be your job." The feeling you get in the pit of your stomach and the weight you feel on your shoulders, that's emotional stress. In the short term this kind of stress can lead to both headache and back ache. Keep that stress up in the long term and it can actually lead to back injury. How? Many people hold their emotional stress in their muscles especially the muscle of the neck, upper and mid back, low back and hips. This stress causes these muscles to tighten and stay tight. Normally blood flows through these muscles but when the muscles are contracted and stay that way the blood flow is impeded, like parking your car on the garden hose. The blood flow is limited or even cut off and when that happens your body sends a pain signal to your brain to let you know all is not well. If these muscles stay tight for long periods of time they can begin to pull the skeletal structure out of alignment causing nerve impingement and other structural issues with the spine causing long term pain and injury. Not good.

Now you may not be able to keep people from stressing you out but you can control the level of your stress. There are several ways to do this. I have put together several techniques that can be very valuable tools in lowering stress while at work. I chose these techniques because they are simple to do, don't attract a lot of attention (no, people won't be standing at the door to your cubicle pointing and giggling) and can be done in just a few minutes. Best of all they work. Try out several of these techniques and see which one works best for you. A word of advice, like most things in life the more you practice these techniques the more adept you get at doing it and the more affective the technique becomes at lowering your stress levels. Practice makes perfect…maybe not perfect but at least pretty darn good.

Body Scan

This stress reduction technique is great because it forces you to redirect your attention. Often we stress ourselves out by thinking about a problem or situation and going through all the negative things that "might" happen. We end up fixated on our problem ramping up our stress levels as we run the negative movie reel over and over in our heads. The Body Scan brings your thoughts inward, focusing your mind on how your body feels and away from the perceived problem. It also asks you to take action against the stress that is building up inside you.

- Sit in your chair, relax your body and close your eyes.
- Feel your head and skull. Sense its weight. Feel your scalp and forehead allow the muscles in the scalp and forehead to relax.
- Feel your eyes. Sense if there is tension in your eyes. Sense if you are forcibly closing your eyelids. Consciously relax your eyelids and feel the tension slide off the eyes.
- Feel your mouth and jaw. Consciously relax them. Pay particular attention to your jaw muscles and unclench them if you need to. Feel your mouth and jaw relax.
- Feel your neck. Sense its weight. Consciously release the tension in the muscles in the neck, feel your neck relax.
- Feel your shoulders. Sense their weight. Consciously relax the muscles across the tops of the shoulders and all around the shoulder joints. Allow your shoulders to relax.
- Feel your arms and hands. Feel their weight. Relax all the muscles in your arms and hands all the way down to the tips of your fingers. Feel your arms and hands relax.
- Feel your abdomen and chest. Sense your breathing. Consciously will them to relax. Deepen your breathing slightly and feel your abdomen and chest relax.
- Feel your buttocks. Sense their weight. Consciously relax the muscles and feel them release. Allow your buttocks to relax
- Feel your upper legs. Feel their weight. Consciously relax The muscles in the front and back of the thighs and feel the tension drift away.

- Feel the lower legs. Feel their weight. Consciously relax the muscles of the calves and lower legs. Feel the lower legs relax.
- Feel your feet. Sense their weight. Consciously relax them. Start with your ankles and progress to your toes. Feel your feet relax.\
- Mentally scan your body. If you find any place that is still tense, then consciously relax that place. Now feel your entire body grow heavy and slowly sink down towards the earth beneath you.

Slowly open your eyes and become aware of your surroundings. Take a moment to become aware of how you feel now compared to how you felt when you began the visualization. Remember that meditation is a practice. If you found this difficult or could not concentrate, don't give up. Continue to do this on a regular basis, and you will soon find that it will become easier and more effective allowing you to become more focused and obtain a deeper sense of relaxation.

Toes Progressive Relaxation

Toes Progressive Relaxation brings focus, physical movement and breath control to the equation of stress relief. By contracting and relaxing the toes you effectively give yourself a foot massage (ok it's not exactly a foot massage but the closest thing to it you'll get at the office). You're also slowing your breathing which helps calm the nervous system. Lay on your back, close your eyes.

- Bring your awareness to your toes.
- Now pull all 10 toes back toward you. Count to 10 slowly.
- Now relax your toes.
- Begin to inhale slowly through your nose if possible. Fill the lower part of your chest first, then the middle and top

part of your chest and lungs. Be sure to do this slowly, over 8 to 10 seconds.

- Now hold your breath for a few seconds
- Slowly exhale through your mouth making a whoosh noise
- Now pull all 10 toes back toward you. Count to 10 slowly.
- Now relax your toes.
- Begin to inhale slowly. Fill the lower part of your chest first, then the middle and top part of your chest and lungs. Be sure to do this slowly, over 8 to 10 seconds.
- Now hold your breath for a few seconds
- Slowly exhale through your mouth making a whoosh noise
- Now pull all 10 toes back toward you. Count to 10 slowly.
- Now relax your toes.

Full Body Progressive Relaxation

Full body progressive relaxation can be a bit tougher to pull off at work, especially if you have no privacy (like an office or cubicle) but this technique can be especially effective at reducing stress so I'm going to include it.

Find a comfortable seated position and try to relax your body. Slowly inhale through your nose. As you inhale tense all the muscles in and around your face. Tense the muscles of your forehead, purse your lips, tighten your jaw muscles and squeeze your eyes shut. Tighten every muscle of your face and head as tight as you can. Hold your breath for one or two seconds then release the air from your lungs like air escaping a balloon as you relax all the muscles of the face and head at once. Gently shake your head then roll your head in a circle, then reverse the circle.

Slowly inhale through your nose. As you inhale tense all the muscles of your shoulders, arms and chest. Pull your shoulders up towards your head, bring your arms in tight to your sides and squeeze as you ball your hands into tight fists. Tighten every muscle in your shoulders arms and chest as tight as you can. Hold your breath for one or two seconds then release the air from your lungs like air escaping a balloon as you drop your arms down to your sides and relax all the muscles in your shoulders arms and chest. Gently shake the arms then roll the shoulders in a circle. Reverse the roll.

Slowly inhale through your nose. As you inhale tense all the muscles of your lower body. Tighten your butt, your thighs your calves and grip the floor with your toes as tightly as you can. Hold your breath for one or two seconds then release the air from your lungs like air escaping a balloon as you relax all the muscles of your lower body. Gently shake one leg then the other.

Slowly inhale through your nose. As you inhale tense all the muscles of your whole body. Tighten all your muscles as you hold your breath for one or two seconds then release the air from your lungs like air escaping a balloon as you relax all the muscles of your whole body. Gently shake your whole body then roll the head and shoulders.

Bellows Breath

The Bellows Breath is adapted from a yogic breathing technique. Its aim is to raise vital energy and increase alertness.

Inhale and exhale rapidly through your nose, keeping your mouth closed but relaxed. Your breaths in and out should be equal in duration, but as short as possible. This is a noisy breathing exercise.

Try for 3 in-and-out breath cycles per second. This produces a quick movement of the diaphragm, suggesting a bellows. Breathe normally after each cycle.

Do not do for more than 15 seconds on your first try. Each time you practice the Bellows Breath, you can increase your time by 5 seconds or so, until you reach a full minute.

If done properly, you may feel invigorated, comparable to the heightened awareness you feel after a good workout. You should feel the effort at the back of the neck, the diaphragm, the chest and the abdomen. Try this breathing exercise the next time you need an energy boost and feel yourself reaching for a cup of coffee. (From Dr. Andrew Weil's website www.drweil.com)

Alternate Nostril Breathing

Alternate nostril breathing creates optimum function of both sides of the brain, improves mood, strengthens the lungs and energizes the body.

- Close off the right nostril with your right thumb then inhale through the left nostril to a three-count
- Hold your breath for an eight-count
- Release your thumb from your right nostril and exhale through the right nostril for a count of 6 as you close off the left nostril with your left thumb.
- Now inhale through your right nostril for a three-count and repeat this on both sides for 1 to 3 minutes.

4-7-8 Breath

This exercise is utterly simple, takes almost no time, requires no equipment and can be done anywhere. Although you can do the exercise in any position, it is best to sit with your back straight while learning the exercise. Place the tip of your tongue against the ridge of tissue just behind your upper front teeth, and keep it there through the entire exercise. You will be exhaling through your mouth around your tongue; try pursing your lips slightly if this seems awkward.

- Exhale completely through your mouth, making a whoosh sound.
- Close your mouth and inhale quietly through your nose to a mental count of 4.
- Hold your breath for a count of 7.
- Exhale completely through your mouth, making a whoosh sound to a count of 8.

- This is 1 breath. Now inhale again and repeat the cycle 3 more times for a total of 4 breaths. (From Dr. Andrew Weil's website www.drweil.com)

Cooling Breath

This breath is meant to cool the nervous system and mind. This simple breathing technique is a great way to relieve stress and cool down a hot temper.

- Stick your tongue out of your mouth and curl it creating a small "straw-" like tube with the tongue.
- Slowly and smoothly suck air in through the tongue filling the lungs with air. Draw the tongue into the mouth and close the lips.
- Hold the breath for a count of 5, then exhale slowly and smoothly through the nostrils.
- Repeat 3 times.

15
25 Exercises for Back Health to do at Your Desk

To do some of these exercises you will need:

- A pair of hand weights (somewhere between 1-10 lbs., depending upon your strength level)
- Rubber tubing/resistance bands with handles and a tab that allows the band to be anchored safely into a doorway
- An inflatable exercise ball that is the correct diameter for your height

Don't forget the safety notes I gave you earlier about working with resistance bands! And make sure that the band you are using for the exercise has enough resistance that the last 10 seconds of reps are very challenging. This will take a bit of experimentation with the individual exercises and your bands and workstation challenges. Don't get discouraged. And as you get stronger, you'll find that you'll be using the higher resistance bands more than the lower resistance bands.

1. Ball Plank:
Kneel on the floor with the ball in front of you. Place your forearms on the ball making sure that the spine remains long and straight. Tighten your stomach muscles and slowly push forward with your feet letting the ball roll away from you, being sure to keep your arms flexed at the elbows. Keeping the back long and flat, hold your body still as you balance on your forearms on the ball. Hold for 15 seconds then return to starting position. Repeat for 1 minute.

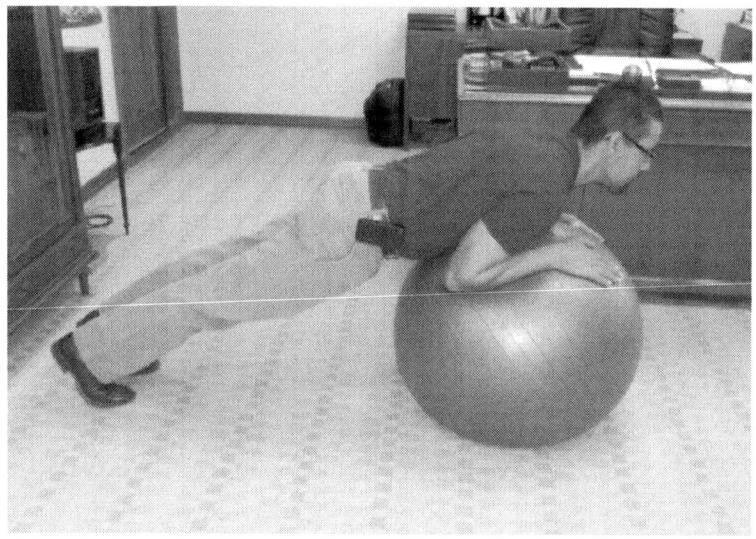

Ball Plank

2. Trunk Extension with Ball:

Kneel on the floor placing the ball under your stomach and hips; your feet should be about shoulder width apart. Bring your hands behind your head as you drape your body over the ball. Slowly raise your torso up off of the ball as far as you can and hold for 15 seconds keeping the ball still beneath you. Return to original position then repeat for 1 minute.

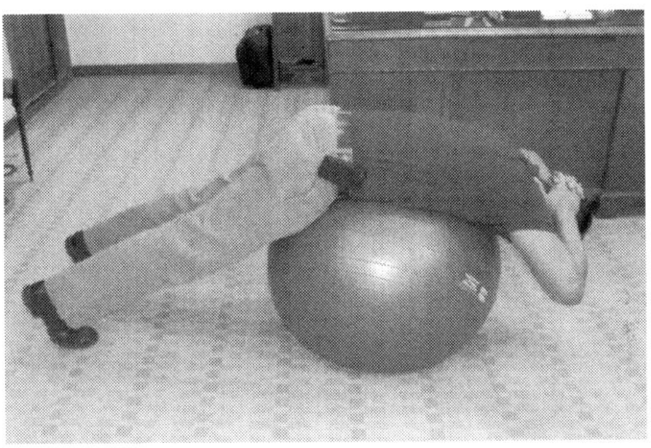

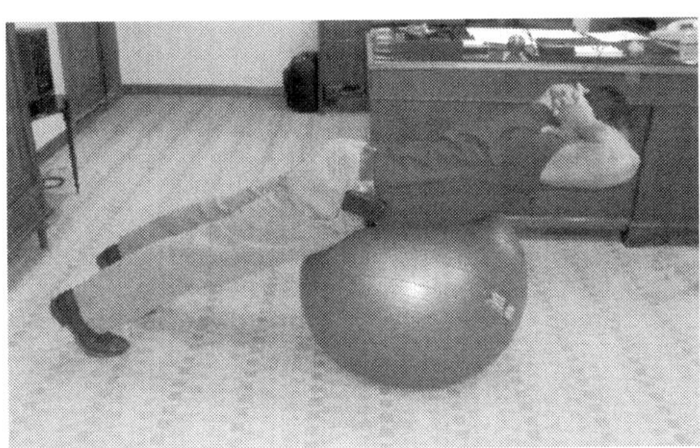

Trunk Extension with Ball

3. Seated Ball Twist with Hand Weights:
Begin in a tall seated position on the ball holding a set of hand weights against your chest. With both feet on the floor, gently turn to the right keeping your spine long, yet relaxed. Without straining your neck, turn your head and torso as if you were going to look behind you. Be sure to keep the ball centered beneath you and steady as you turn from side to side in a slow, controlled manner. Repeat turning from side to side for 1 minute.

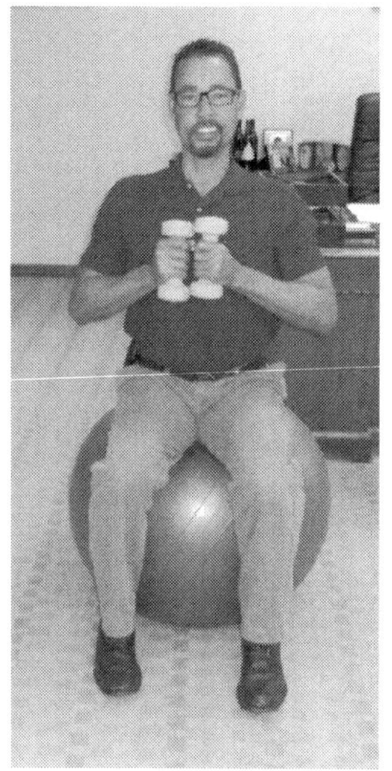

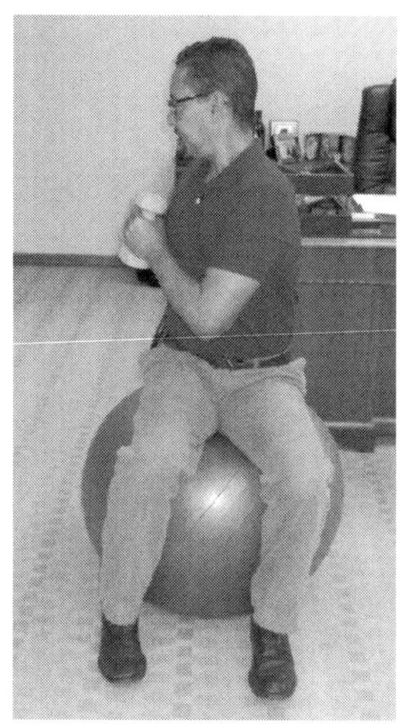

Seated Ball Twist with Hand Weights

4. Ball Sits with Single Arm Raises:

Begin in a tall seated position on the ball with both hands resting on your thighs. Keeping the ball still under you slowly raise one arm high over head as if to touch the ceiling. Then lower that arm and raise the opposite arm. Continue to alternate arms, keeping the ball centered beneath you and as still as possible for 1 minute.

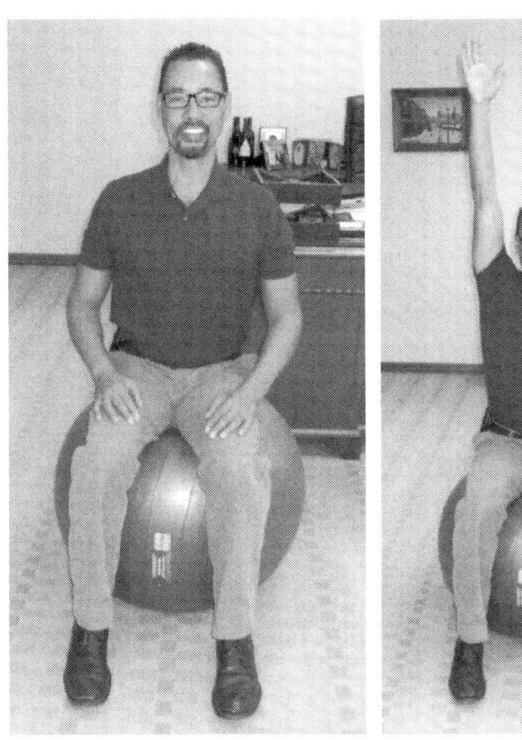
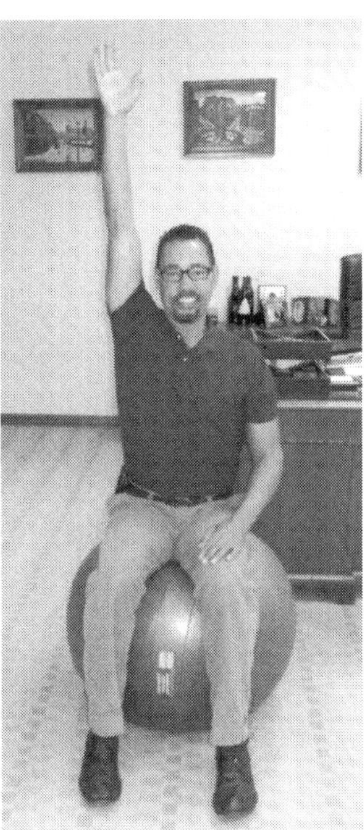

Ball Sits with Single Arm Raises

5. Wood Chopper with Pulse at Top:
Grasp handles of bands in each hand and step on the center portion of the bands. Still standing on the band, step feet out so that they are hip distance apart. Bring hands together and hold both handles at the same time with both hands. Bring both hands to the left side of the body. Pull the band across the body upwards towards the right shoulder and tug upward three times. Return to original position. Repeat for 30 seconds, then switch sides and repeat for 30 seconds.

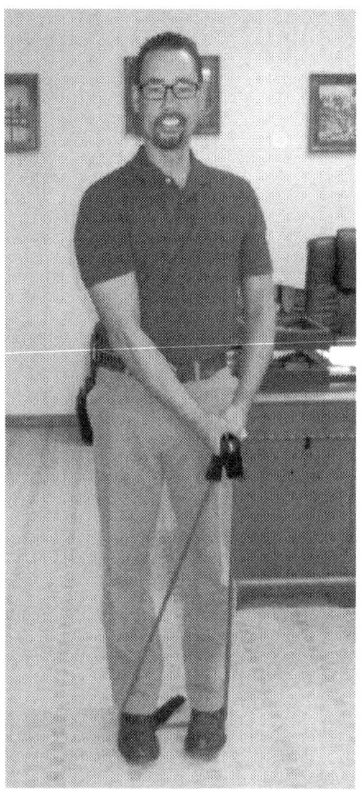
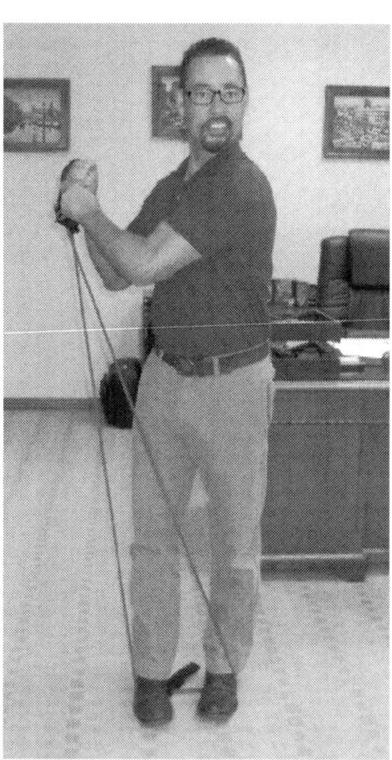

Wood Chopper with Pulse at Top

6. Seated Rows with Resistance Band:
Secure the band in a door or to a stationary object so it will be at chest level while you are seated. Be sure the band is secure and will not release unexpectedly. Facing the anchor point, grasp a handle in each hand and sit far enough from the anchor point that the band is free of slack when your arms are fully extended in front of you. Engage your core, keeping your upper body still and upright. Bring arms back towards your chest, sweeping the elbows out and back until your hands are even with your upper chest. The motion should be similar to the action of rowing a boat with two oars. Repeat for 1 minute.

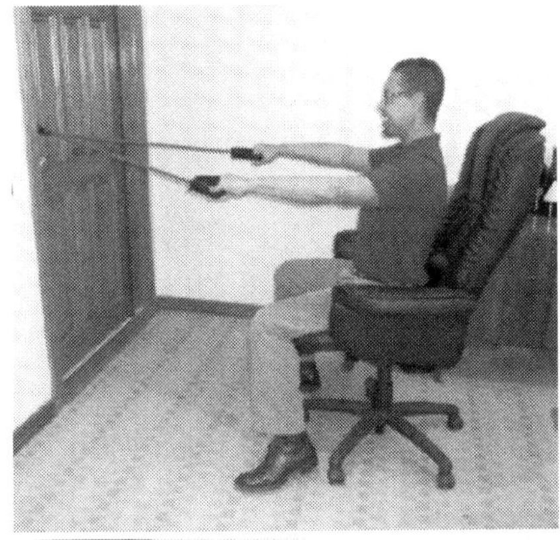

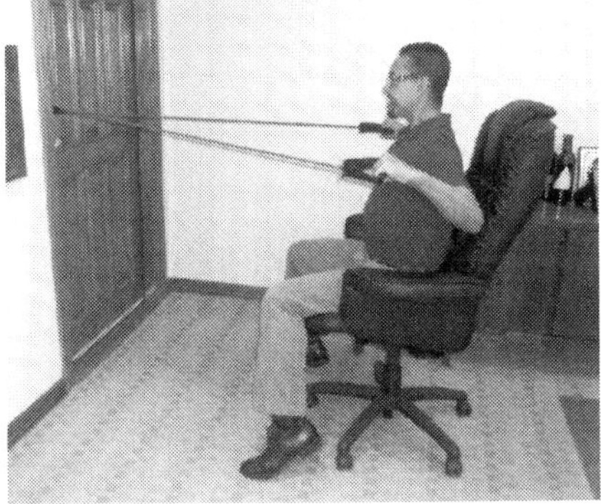

Seated Rows with Resistance Band

7. Twist with Resistance Band:

Attach resistance band into a doorway or other secure object at about chest height while standing. Stand far enough from the connection point that the band is taught and has no slack in it. Hold the handles of the band at chest height then slowly turn the torso and shoulders away from the attachment point, twisting at the hips, but keeping the feet still. Return to starting position and repeat for 30 seconds. Then switch sides.

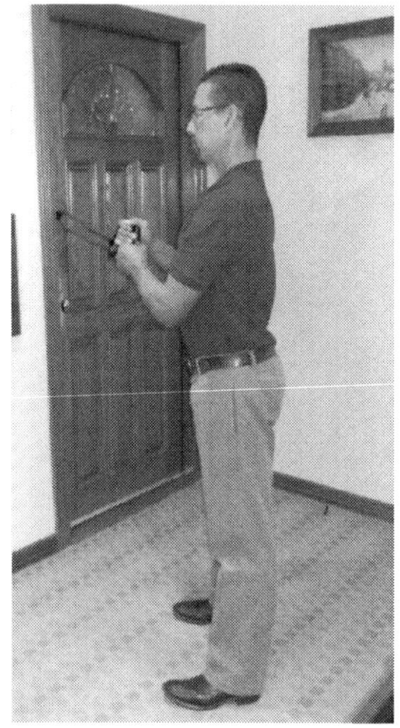

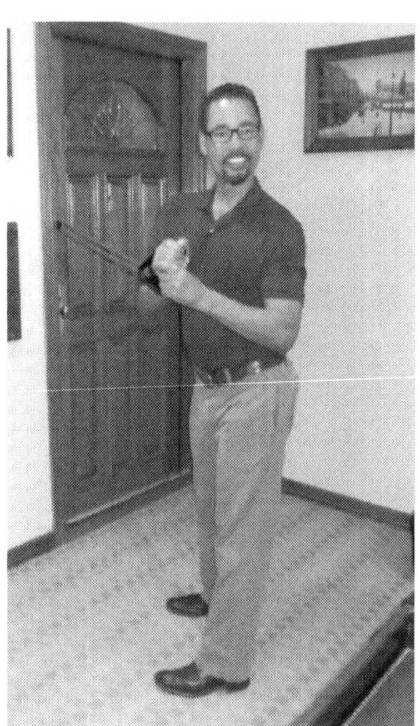

Twist with Resistance Band

8. Hip Flexor Stretch:

Stand and hold onto a chair or your desk with your left hand. Bend your right knee, bringing your right heel up towards your buttocks. Reach down and grab your right ankle. Pull your knee cap down towards the floor and press your right hip gently forward. Hold for 30 seconds. Switch sides.

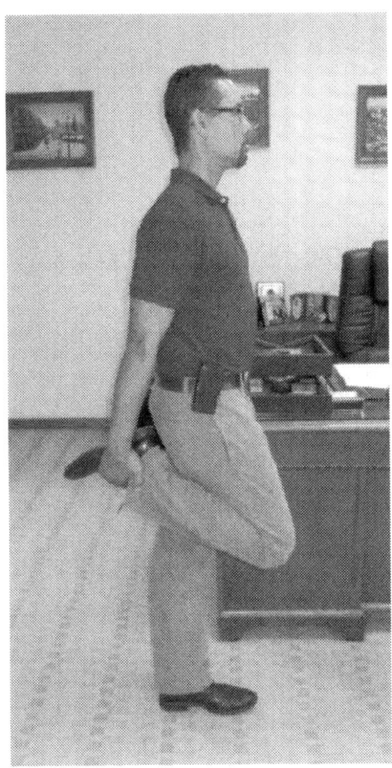
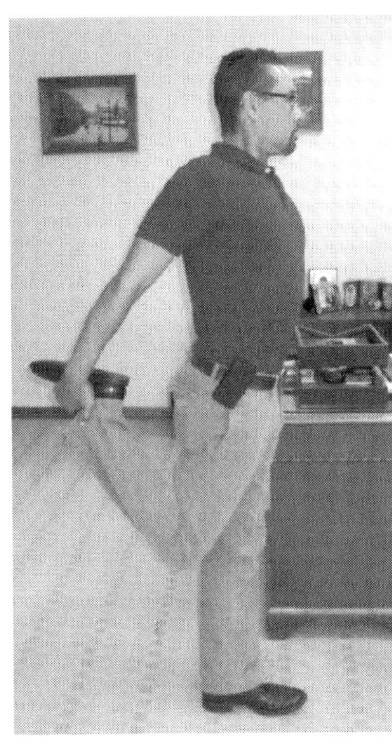

Hip Flexor Stretch

9. Hamstring Stretch:

From a standing position step forward with your right foot approximately 2 feet, keeping your right knee straight but not locked. Hinge at the hips, leaning forward until you feel a gentle stretch in the back of the right thigh. Hold for 30 seconds and switch legs.

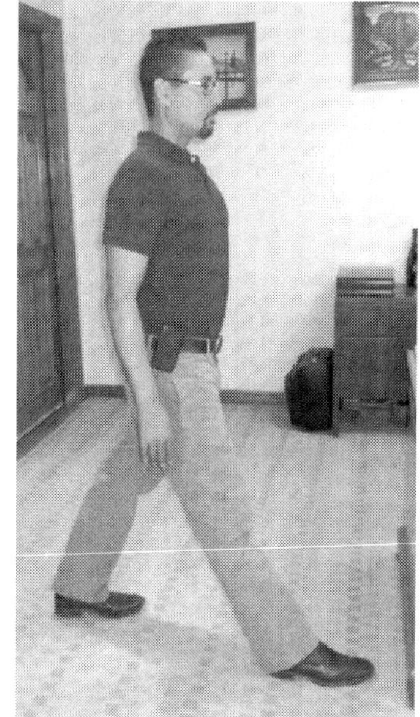

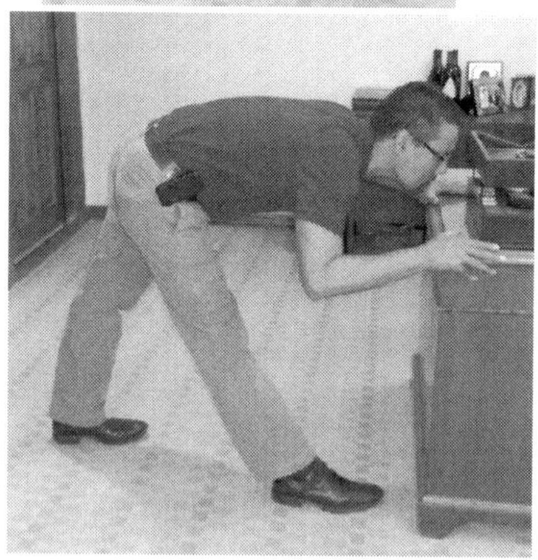

Hamstring Stretch

10. Toppling Tree:

Stand and hold onto a chair or your desk with your left hand. Bend your right knee bringing your right heel up towards your buttocks. Reach down and grab your right ankle (If you have trouble grasping your ankle you can use a strap or rubber tubing). Pull your knee back and away from your body and press your right hip gently forward as you lean forward and bring your torso up and look forward. Hold for 30 seconds. Switch sides.

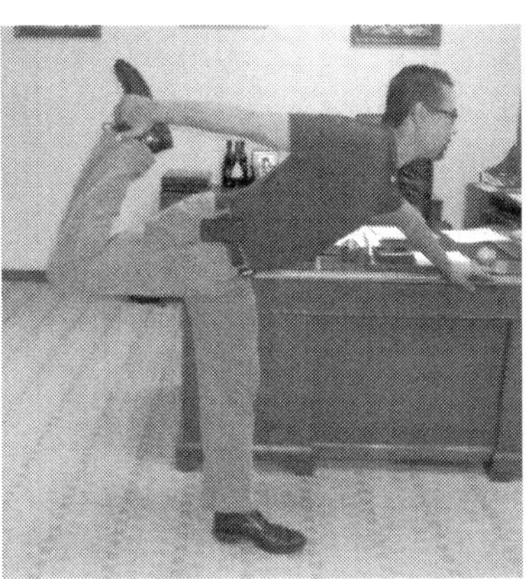

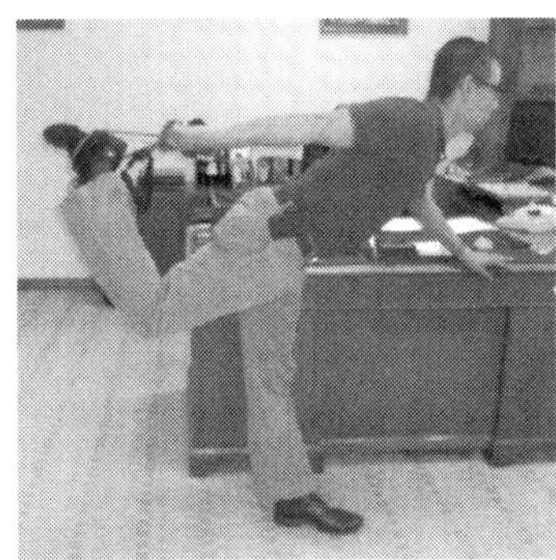

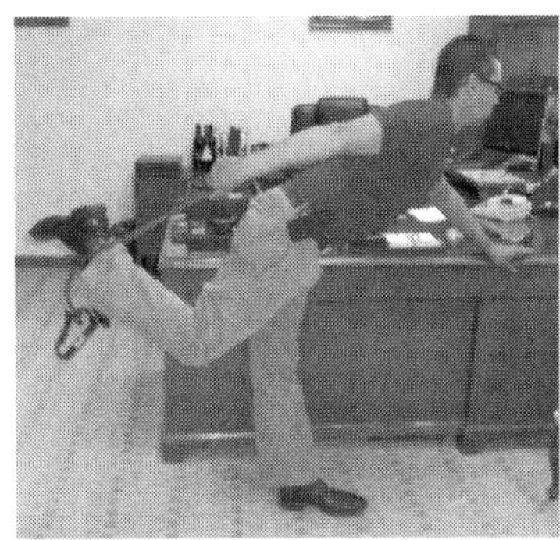

Toppling Tree (with Modifications)

11. Sitting Man Style Stretch:

Begin in a tall seated position. Cross your right ankle over your left knee, creating a triangle shape with your right leg, then gently press down on the inside of your right knee until you feel a gentle stretch through the hip and buttocks. Hold for 30 seconds. Now gently lean forward, bringing the chest down towards the legs; this should intensify the stretch. Hold for another 30 seconds. Switch sides and repeat on the other side, then return to your tall seated position.

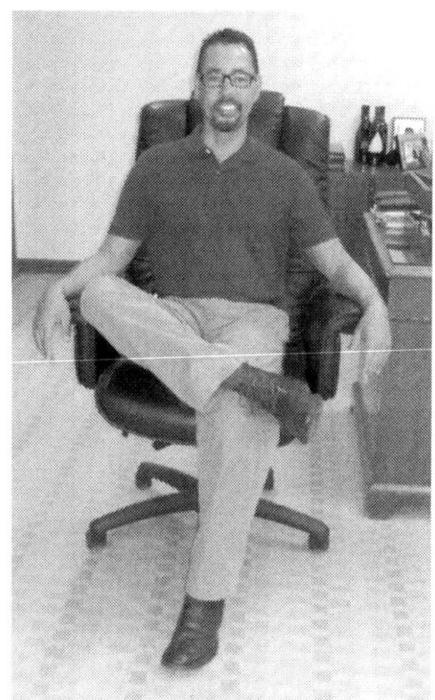

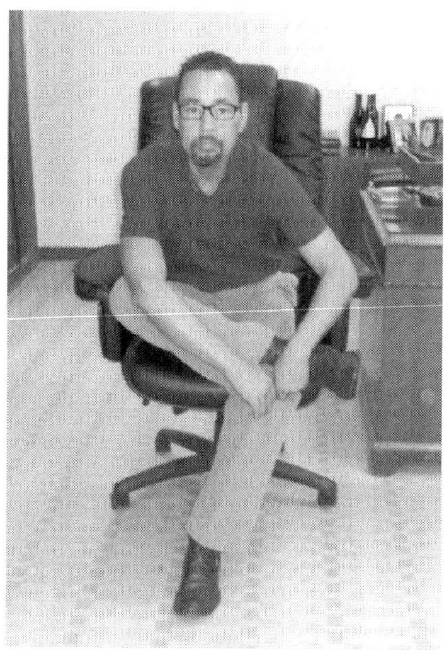

Sitting Man Style Stretch

12. Standing Spine Stabilizer:

Stand in front of a desk or chair that will not move, at arm's length distance from the object. Lean forward and place both hands on it for stabilization. Leaning on the desk, slowly raise your right arm and reach forward as far as you can at the same time lift your left foot off the floor reaching back with that foot as far as you can. Be sure to keep your hips square with the floor beneath you as you balance on your right leg and try to keep as little weight on your left hand as possible. Hold for 30 seconds and repeat on opposite side.

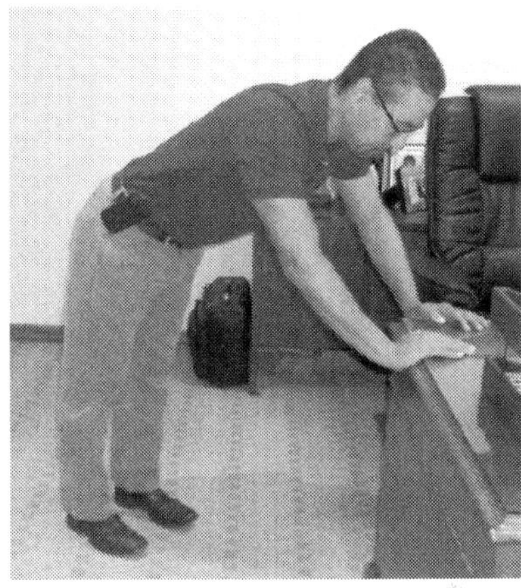

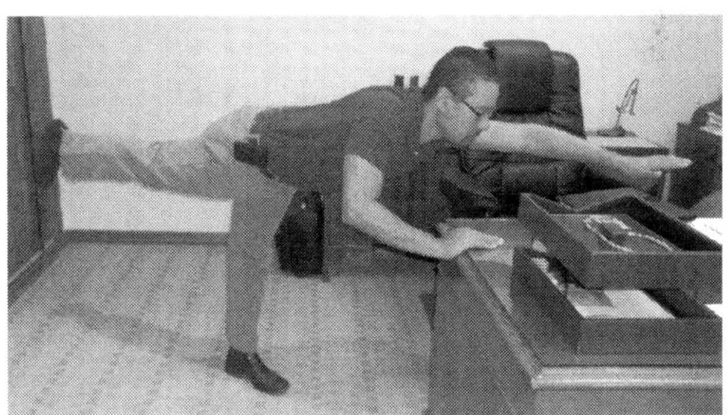

Standing Spine Stabilizer

13. Roll Down and Roll up:
Stand up tall with your back to a wall, heels six to eight inches from the wall. Slowly drop your chin down to your chest then one vertebra at a time slowly roll down as you work on flexibility and articulation of the spine. You should end up with your hands on your thighs with your head down in a hanging position. From the hanging position, reverse the action you did with roll down and slowly roll up stacking your vertebrae one atop the other from the bottom up until you are once again standing tall against the wall. Repeat for one minute.

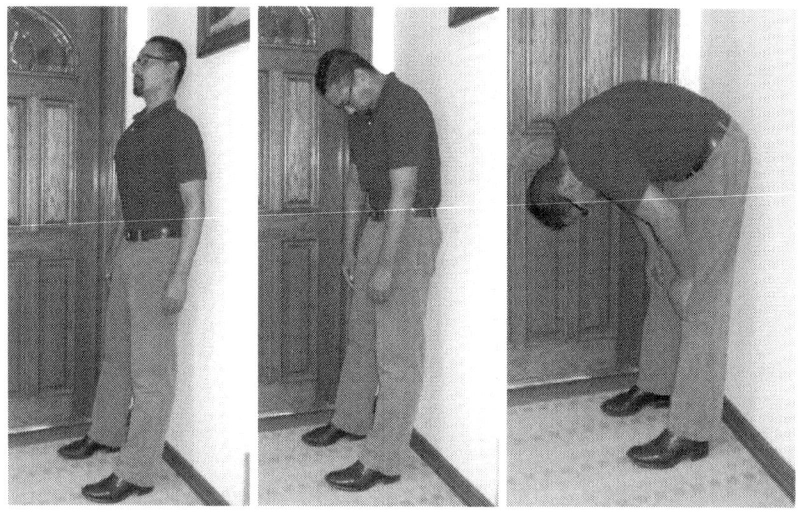

Roll Down and Roll Up

14. Shoulder Blade Squeeze:

Standing tall with the feet hip distance apart, begin by rolling the shoulders forward and making your back as wide as possible. Then pull the shoulder blades together squeeze tightly then roll the shoulder blades down as you pull the shoulders down and away from the ears. Be sure to keep the spine tall and straight throughout the exercise. Roll the shoulders forward again and repeat the sequence for 30 seconds.

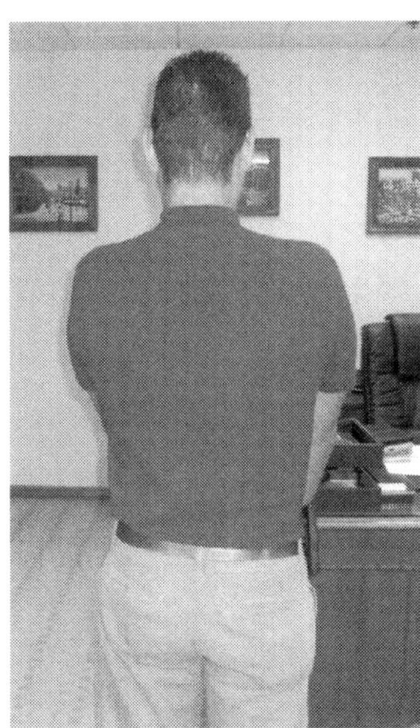

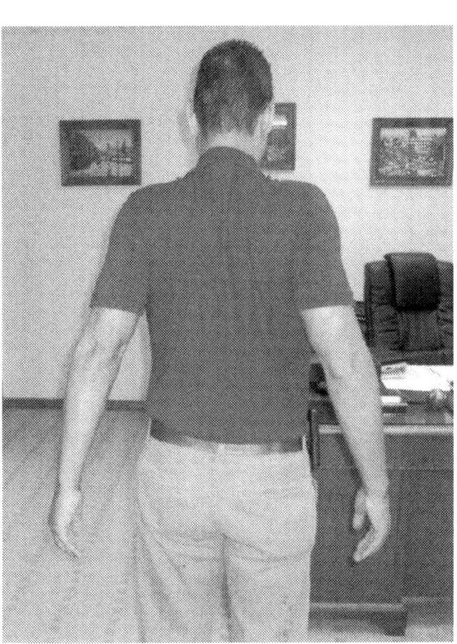

Shoulder Blade Squeeze

15. Powerful Pose:

Stand with feet hip distance apart and reach with both hands up towards the sky, keeping the hands shoulder width apart. Bend the knees and drop the buttocks down as if you were going to sit in a chair. Lengthen the spine until your head feels like it is floating away from your tailbone but continue to look forward not up. Hold for 30 seconds.

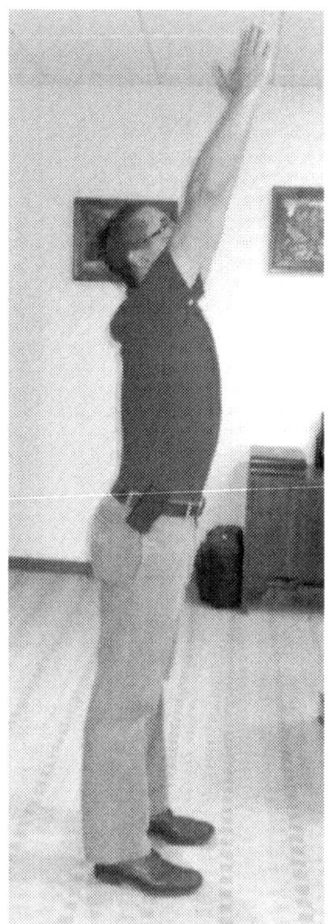
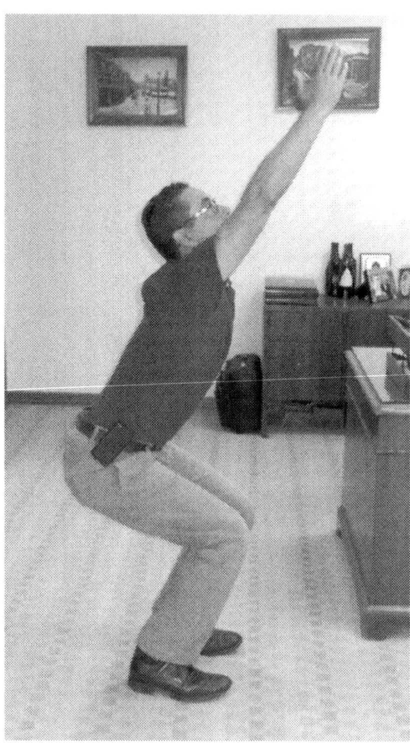

Powerful Pose

16. Seated Chair Twist:

Begin in a tall seated position. With both feet on the floor, gently turn to the right keeping your spine long, yet relaxed. With your right arm, reach to the back of your chair as you twist the torso using the back of the chair as leverage. Without straining your neck, turn your head and torso as if you were going to look behind you. Hold for 30 seconds. Repeat on the opposite side. Return to your tall seated position.

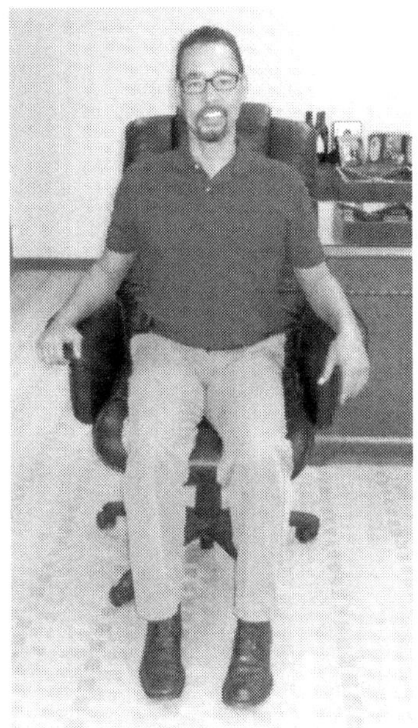

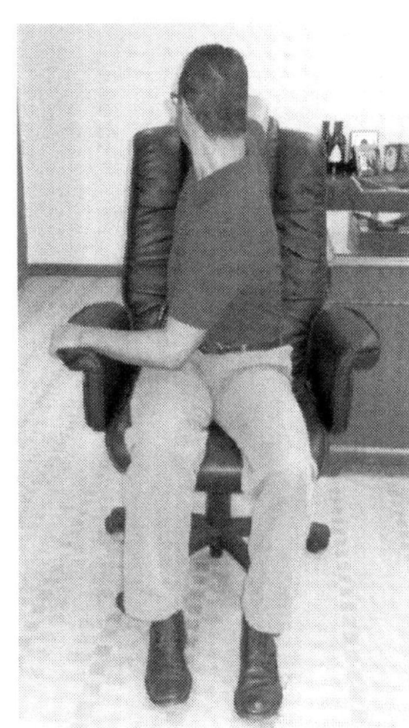

Seated Chair Twist

17. Turning the Head:

Begin in a standing position with arms hanging at your sides and the palms of your hands facing your body. *Very slowly* turn your head to the right and look over your right shoulder as you rotate the palms of your hands out so that they point out and away from your body. *Very slowly* turn your head back so that you are looking forward again as you rotate your palms back so that they face your body again. *Very slowly* turn your head to the left and look over your left shoulder as you rotate your palms out so that they point out and away from your body. *Very slowly* turn your head back so that you are looking forward again as you rotate your palms back so that they face your body again. Repeat for 30 seconds.

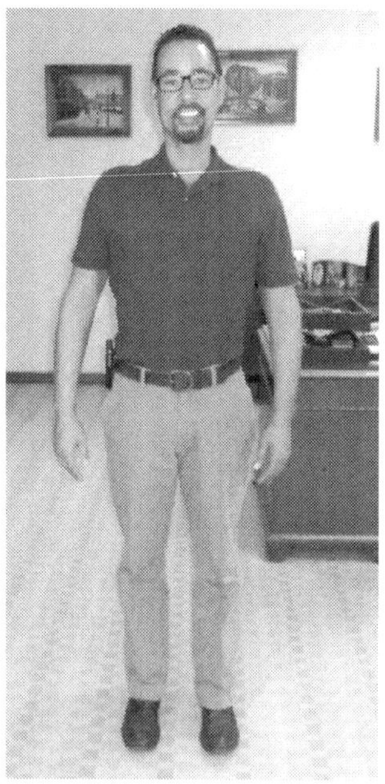

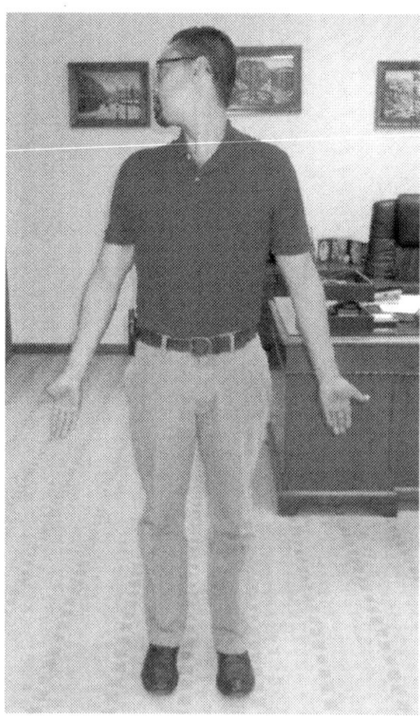

Turning the Head

18. Baby Camel Prays to the Gods:

From a standing position place your hands on the front of your thighs for support, then lean forward as you roll your shoulders inward and round the back, dropping your chin down to your chest creating a humped back. Pause for a moment, and then one vertebra at a time bring yourself back up to your standing position bringing your arms down to your sides. Slowly roll your shoulders back, lift the chest and look to the sky. Repeat for one minute.

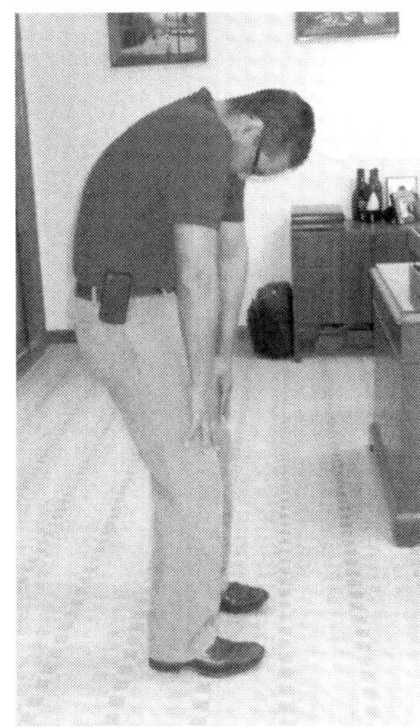

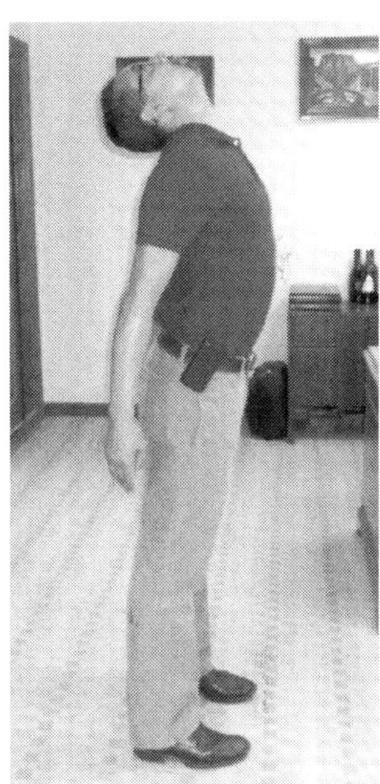

Baby Camel Prays to the Gods

19. Hip Swivels:

Stand with your feet hip distance apart. Place your hands on your hips and slowly start to roll your hips in a circle. With each swivel of your hips make the circles a little bigger. After 10 seconds, switch directions.

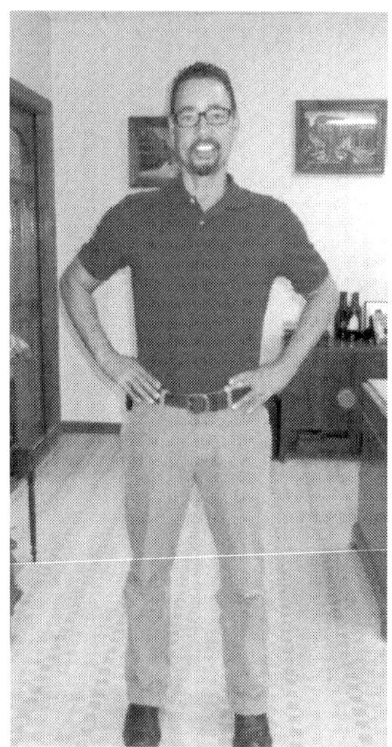

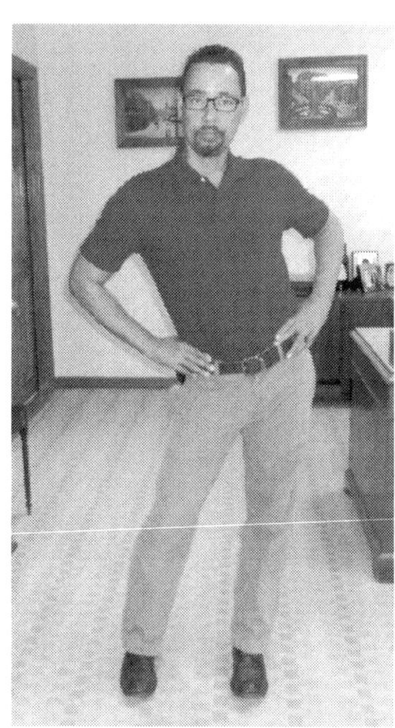

Hip Swivels

20. Bending Backwards:
Begin by standing in front of a stable desk or chair that will not move. Turn your back to the desk or chair and place the palms of your hands on the desk or chair behind you with your fingers pointed away from your body. Keeping your hands on the desk or chair, take a short step away with both feet, then arch your back and press your chest up towards the ceiling. Gently drop your head back and look up at the ceiling. Hold for 30 seconds and then walk your feet back to the original position.

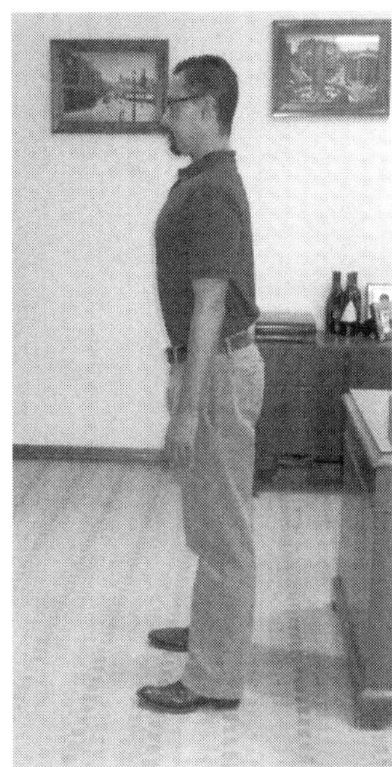
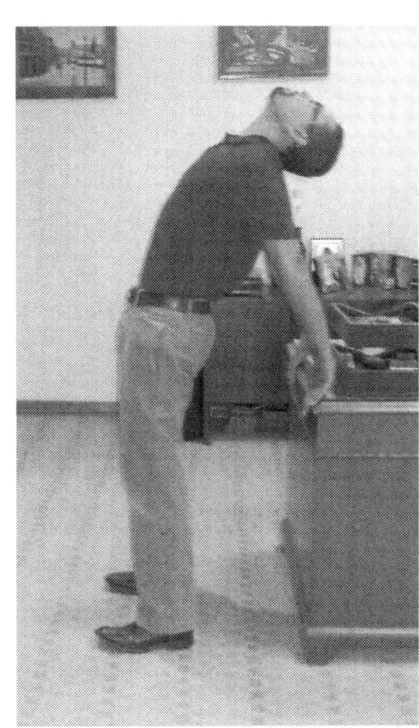

Bending Backwards

21. Wide Leg Chair Squats:

Begin by sitting on a chair with feet wider than hip distance apart and toes pointed outward. Your knees should be aligned directly over your ankles. Sit up tall and bring your arms out in front of you at shoulder height with the palms of your hands pointed in towards the center line of your body. Stand, then drop the buttocks down as if to sit, trying to keep as much weight *off* the chair as you can when coming down to the seated position. Press back up to the original position. Repeat for one minute.

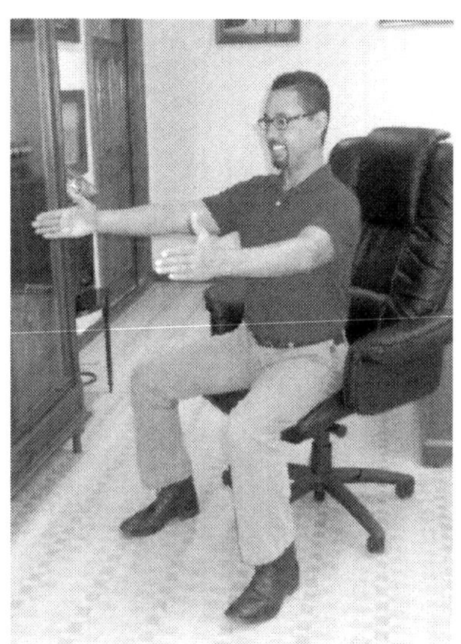
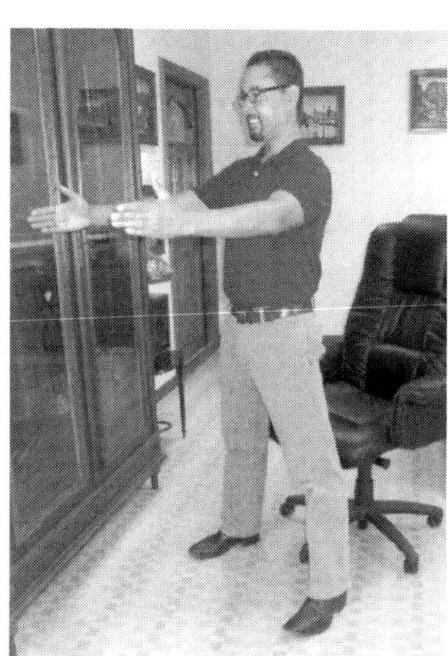

Wide Leg Chair Squats

22. Forward Fold:
Begin in a standing position with feet hip distance apart. Bend both knees slightly, then lean forward and slowly lower your head as you begin to reach down toward your mid-thighs or knees depending on what feels comfortable for you. Support the upper body with your hands, and allow the spine to lengthen toward the floor as much as feels comfortable. Hold this pose for 30 seconds.

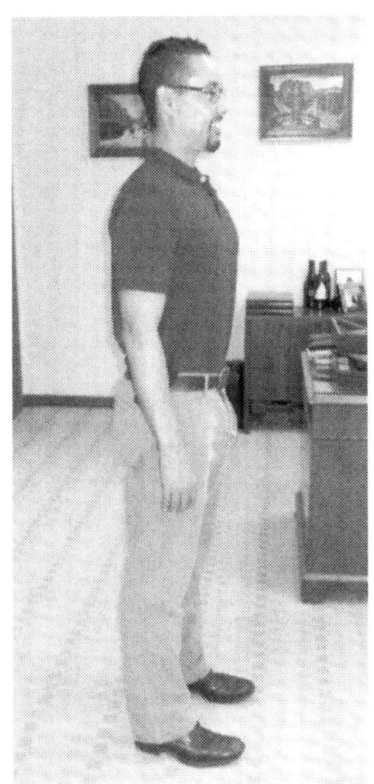

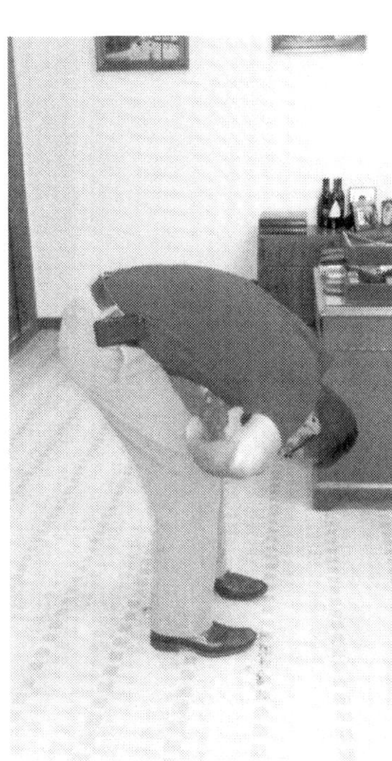

Forward Fold

23. Round and Open:
Sitting in a chair with your feet on the floor, begin by bringing your shoulders directly above your hips, lengthening your spine upward as your head floats away from your shoulders. Drop your chin down to your chest and slowly lean forward as you roll the shoulders in towards the chest, making an exaggerated hump in your back. Bring your forearms to the fronts of your thighs as you pull the shoulder blades apart. Hold for 30 seconds as you breathe. Now, slowly, one vertebra at a time, bring yourself back up to a tall seated position, then roll your shoulders back, open the chest, arch the back and look up to the ceiling. Breathe deeply as you let your arms drop down to your sides. Hold for 30 seconds and come back to the tall seated position.

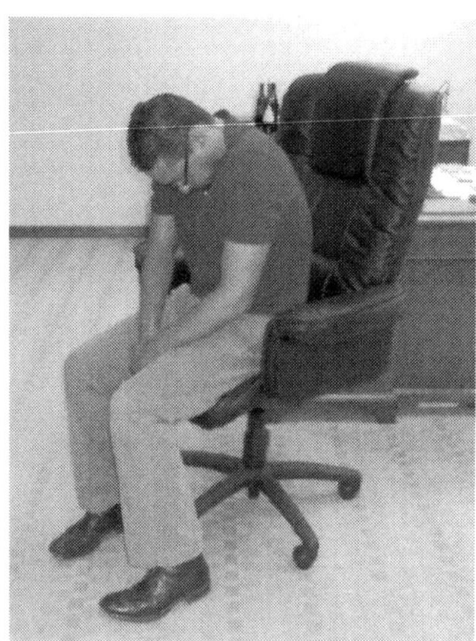

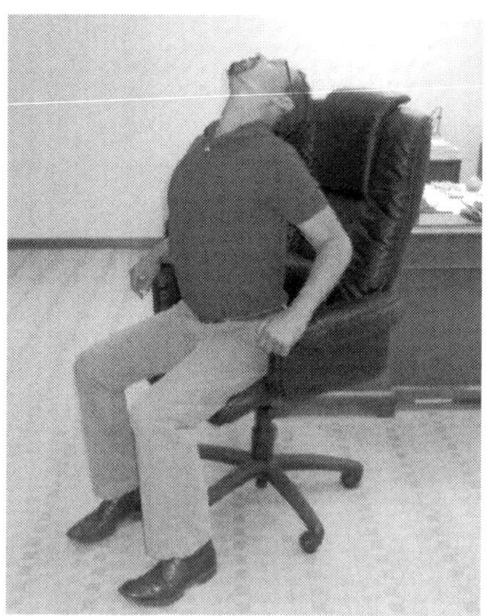

Round and Open

24. Incline Leg Pull Down:

Stand 3 to 4 feet from a desk or table that will not move and can support your weight. Bring yourself into push-up position with your hands on the desk or wall and your feet on the floor. Hands should be directly below the shoulders and the spine should be long, making sure that your hips don't sag or your bottom isn't sticking up in the air; your body should be angled from the ground to the desk. Keeping your core engaged and your butt down, press your left foot firmly into the ground and lift your right foot as high as you can without opening your hip. Hold the foot up for 30 seconds. Bring your right foot back down and then press your right foot firmly into the ground and lift your left foot as high as you can and hold it for 30 seconds. Bring your left foot down.

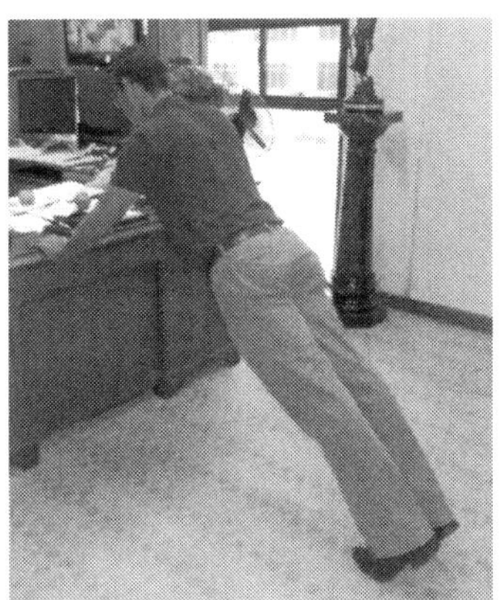

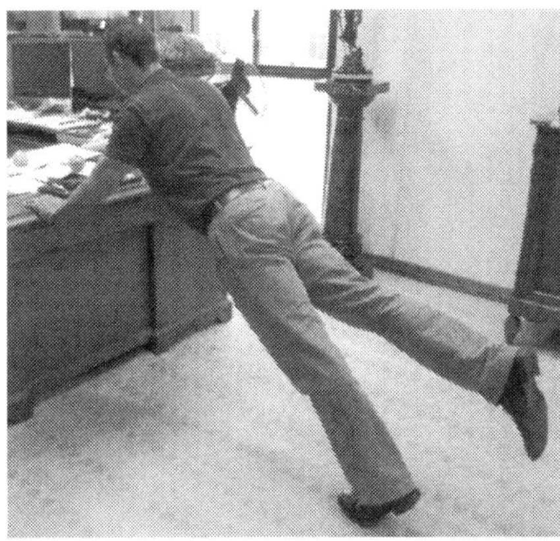

Incline Leg Pull Down

25. Seated Forward Fold:

Sitting in a chair with your feet on the floor with legs spread wide, and hands on knees, hinge at the hips and begin to lean forward. You can leave your hands on your knees, or for a deeper stretch, reach down and grab your lower legs or ankles as you drop the head down towards the floor. Lengthen your spine as if you were increasing the distance between the crown of your head and your tailbone. Hold for one minute, then bring the hands back to the knees and one vertebra at a time, slowly rise back to the upright seated position.

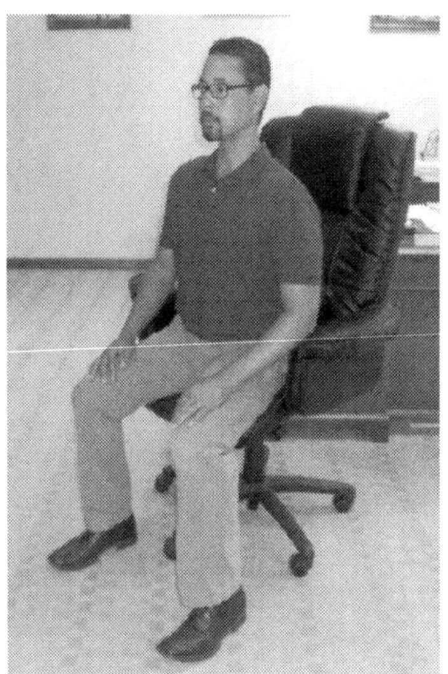

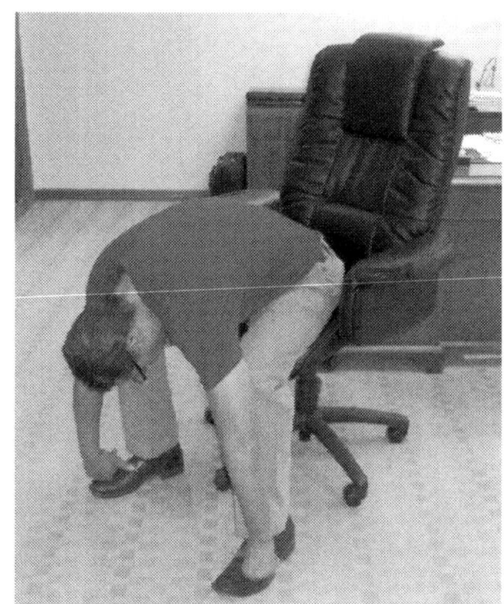

Seated Forward Fold

16
The Back Health Program and Other Programs

I have created a sample three day back health program for the office. This program was designed for people who only want to work on back health. For those of you who are new to this type of training, you may wonder why I am only recommending 3 days of training per week. I do this because it is important to allow the muscles to rest between training sessions. This allows the muscles to grow and allows the body to recover. In a perfect world, you would give yourself one full day of "rest" between training sessions. Having said that, few of us live in perfect worlds, and working out back to back days shouldn't do any harm. But remember that rest is equally as important as the workout. Having said that some of the exercises in this program are flexibility exercises, these exercises can be done daily (I actually recommend doing them daily).

In order to be sure you stay on schedule, just set an alarm on your smart phone or on your daily Outlook calendar to remind you it's time for your 5 minute workout. You'll notice in the "schedules" below that I have you doing your workout at 45 minutes past the hour; that was entirely arbitrary. Create the schedule that works best for you and your workplace. Just keep in mind that you really need to get up and get moving each and every hour.

Each of the exercises listed below should be done for exactly one minute. If you decide to do all five exercises each hour, you should be back to work after no more than five minutes. (If you are pressed for time in any given hour, just do 2 or 3 of the exercises and get back to work!)

Day 1

9:45

- Ball Plank
- Hamstring Stretch
- Wide Leg Chair Squats
- Seated Forward Fold
- Incline Leg Pull Down

10:45

- Hip Swivels
- Wide Leg Chair Squats
- Turning the Head
- Powerful Pose
- Sitting Man Style Stretch

11:45

- Standing Spine Stabilizer
- Seated Chair Twist
- Shoulder Blade Squeeze
- Forward Fold
- Toppling Tree

1:45

- Hip Flexor Stretch
- Twist with Resistance Band
- Baby Camel Prays to the Gods
- Trunk Extension with Ball
- Round and Open

2:45

- Ball Sits with Arm Raises
- Bending Backwards
- Wood Chopper with Pulse
- Hip Swivels
- Seated Ball Twist with Hand Weights

Day 2

10:45

- Hip Flexor Stretch
- Seated Row with Resistance Bands
- Sitting Man Style Stretch
- Shoulder Blade Squeeze
- Turning the Head

11:45

- Wood Chopper with Pulse at Top
- Baby Camel Prays to the Gods
- Toppling Tree
- Hamstring Stretch
- Twist with Resistance Bands

1:45

- Roll Down Roll Up
- Standing Spine Stabilizer
- Seated Chair Twist
- Ball Sits with Single Arm Raises
- Round and Open

2:45

- Incline Leg Pull Down
- Forward Fold
- Wide Leg Chair Squats
- Bending Backwards
- Wood Chopper with Pulse at Top

3:45

- Hip Flexor Stretch
- Ball Plank
- Sitting Man Style
- Seated Ball Twist with Hand Weights
- Hamstring Stretch

Day 3

9:45

- Trunk Extension with Ball
- Seated Forward Fold
- Wood Chopper with Pulse at Top
- Baby Camel Prays to the Gods
- Powerful Pose

10:45

- Seated Chair Twist
- Standing Spine Stabilizer
- Roll Down Roll Up
- Shoulder Blade Squeeze
- Round and Open

11:45

- Seated Rows with Resistance Bands
- Turning the Head
- Ball Plank
- Hip Swivels
- Wide Leg Chair Squats

1:45

- Bending Backwards
- Seated Ball Twists with Hand Weights
- Hip Flexor Stretch
- Toppling Tree
- Sitting Man Style Stretch

2:45

- Incline Leg Pull Down
- Forward Fold
- Twist with Resistance Band
- Hamstring Stretch
- Powerful Pose

5-Day Full Body Program

Day 1

9:45	5 one minute Upper Body Exercises
10:45	5 one minute Lower Body Exercises
11:45	5 one minute Upper Body Exercises
1:45	5 one minute Lower Body Exercises
2:45	5 one minute Upper Body Exercises
3:45	5 one minute Lower Body Exercises

Day 2

9:45	5 one minute Back Health Exercises
10:45	5 one minute Back Health Exercises
11:45	5 one minute Back Health Exercises
1:45	5 one minute Back Health Exercises
2:45	5 one minute Back Health Exercises
3:45	5 one minute Back Health Exercises

Day 3

9:45	5 one minute Lower Body Exercises
10:45	5 one minute Upper Body Exercises
11:45	5 one minute Lower Body Exercises
1:45	5 one minute Upper Body Exercises
2:45	5 one minute Lower Body Exercises
3:45	5 one minute Upper Body Exercises

Day 4

9:45	5 one minute Back Health Exercises
10:45	5 one minute Back Health Exercises
11:45	5 one minute Back Health Exercises
1:45	5 one minute Back Health Exercises
2:45	5 one minute Back Health Exercises
3:45	5 one minute Back Health Exercises

Day 5

9:45	5 one minute Upper Body Exercises
10:45	5 one minute Lower Body Exercises
11:45	5 one minute Upper Body Exercises
1:45	5 one minute Lower Body Exercises
2:45	5 one minute Upper Body Exercises
3:45	5 one minute Lower Body Exercises

17
Conclusion

Clearly being more active is something that would benefit all of us, but the old version of what active means is quickly being wiped away. While changing the way you think can often be difficult and even painful I think that the new reality of being active is a far better way of living and working and in the long run will not only improve the health of our workforce but also improve the health of our businesses.

At the beginning of this book we went over how to use this book as a whole to improve your overall health and wellbeing. Then we learned the "etiquette" of the office workout and how it differs from working out in the gym or in private. Staying within these guidelines will help you keep peace and harmony in the workplace as you improve your health. We also discussed the benefits for you and your employer of bringing more activity to the work day and all of the latest research which demonstrates the health and financial benefits that could result from working out at work. Then we got into the nuts and bolts of how to create a more active work day that is much healthier for your entire body.

Finally we introduced the 75 exercises and sample workout programs you can try in the office.

By implementing the simple strategies in this book you can greatly reduce your risk of developing heart disease, diabetes, certain types of cancer and obesity and have a stronger, more flexible, and healthier back. People who move the most during the day have been shown to have significantly smaller waistlines than their counterparts who sat more often regardless of how much conventional exercise they did. This evidence and much more points to the fact that we should all be doing *The Office Workout*.

So what are you waiting for?

If you liked this book, tell the world! We would really appreciate a review on the book's page at Amazon.com.

Other books by Kent Burden:

Is Your Chair Killing You?

Exercise Sucks! The Secret to Losing Weight Without Really Trying

43787346R00102

Made in the USA
San Bernardino, CA
27 December 2016